Lloyd.

A Journey Of Courage.

A true Story taken from the diaries
Of Lloyd's Mum.

Elaine Beverley Pike.

Contents:

Acknowledgements.

For and on behalf of Lloyd Michael Pike, born 31/10/1991. And I, his mum, Elaine, wish to thank everyone involved with and around Lloyd.

His family, friends, and neighbours. The University Hospital of Wales (Cardiff), Llandough Hospital (Penarth), Velindre Hospital (Cardiff), The Community Nurses of Wales, and Ty Hafan Children's Hospice (Sully).

Thank you all for the kind support and attention you gave to Lloyd.

Lloyd touched the hearts of everyone he met.

He was a brave little soldier.

XXXXXXXXXX

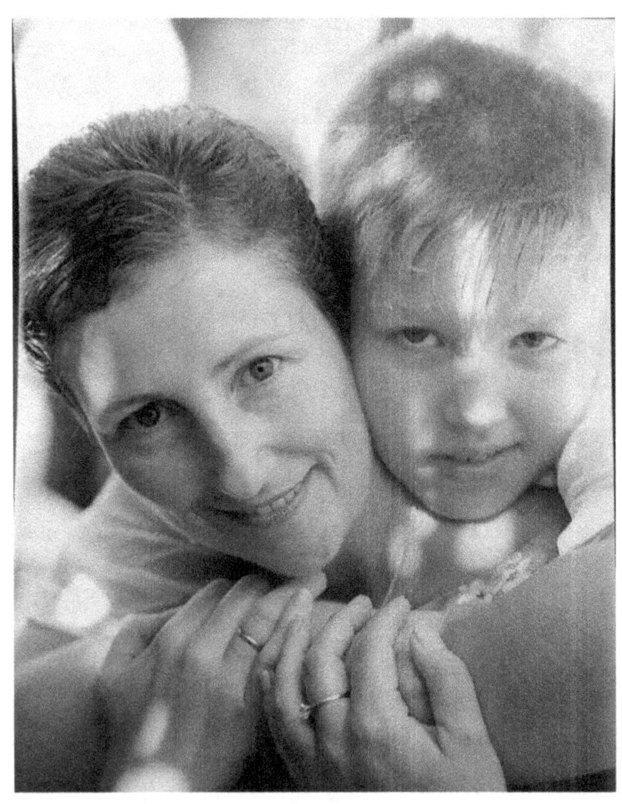

Foreword

This book is about the journey of one of God's lent children.

It is a true story taken from the diaries of a grieving mother and not written by a professional writer. So please excuse the grammar.

Lloyd Michael Pike was born on 31 October 1991 at the Royal Gwent Hospital in Newport, South Wales, and he was a special gift of life for me, Lloyd's mum, Elaine.

I need to let everyone know about Lloyd, as he would want to help people as much as possible. And so this book is my chance to tell everyone about Lloyd's courageous journey.

In 1998, I began noticing Lloyd's illness when he was seven.

They diagnosed Lloyd with a rare brain tumour known as a Pilocytic Astrocytoma, which the surgeons discovered after a biopsy on 3 August 2000, was malignant and inoperable.

Through the book, you will read about Lloyd's journey of courage during operations, MRI scans, chemotherapy, and radiotherapy.

At the end of Lloyd's journey, he spent most of his time with me, his mother, at Ty Hafan Children's Hospice, which Lloyd loved.

It's a very tranquil place, and it was here that Lloyd passed away with his close family in attendance.

Further in the book, I will tell you about our experience with Lloyd's passing, life after Lloyd's death and how we still feel we are together.

Remember, you are not alone.

Chapter One.

A Gift from God.

I, Mum, had been waiting a long time to have news that I was pregnant. And after three years of trying, it was the best news a woman could have had.

My pregnancy was perfect, and I was blooming. I have never felt so happy.

Then, on 31 October 1991, my special little boy, Lloyd Michael Pike, was born. He was 7lb 14ozs, delivered into the world by forceps.

When they placed Lloyd on my stomach, I felt privileged because I am a mother, and I intend to love and cherish Lloyd, giving him the best of everything with all my love and attention.

Being a mum came so naturally to me. The bond between us is staggering. And as any mum will tell you, it is uplifting when you see your flesh and blood crawling, talking, and laughing.

Lloyd had a fantastic smile.

He was a content baby as he progressed in life, and we spent every minute of the day together, which was great because I had been made redundant from my job.

It's brilliant for me to know that I could spend all my time with my baby.

Lloyd's birthdays were great fun. His first was in our house, with all the toddlers around the table in their high chairs.

Lloyd's second birthday party was at a leisure centre that had a bouncy castle. All his birthday parties were fabulous, and I would always be extravagant. Christmas was always a terrific time.

They were all fantastic times.

At Easter, we would do an Easter egg hunt. Even Valentine's Day was special. All occasions were brilliant because Lloyd was an exceptional child.

And such a gorgeous little lad. His chubby cheeks and blonde curly hair are like an angel, although he was born on Halloween, and some people would joke and say he was my little devil.

Not my Lloyd. He is a little angel in my eyes and always will be.

As our life went on and Lloyd went to playgroup, I was always with him, helping and never leaving his side. And then, a couple of years on, it was time for nursery school.

Because I wasn't working, I volunteered to help at the nursery, only so I could be with Lloyd. It worked out fine.

I would help on nursery trips and do anything to help as long as I could be with my Lloyd.

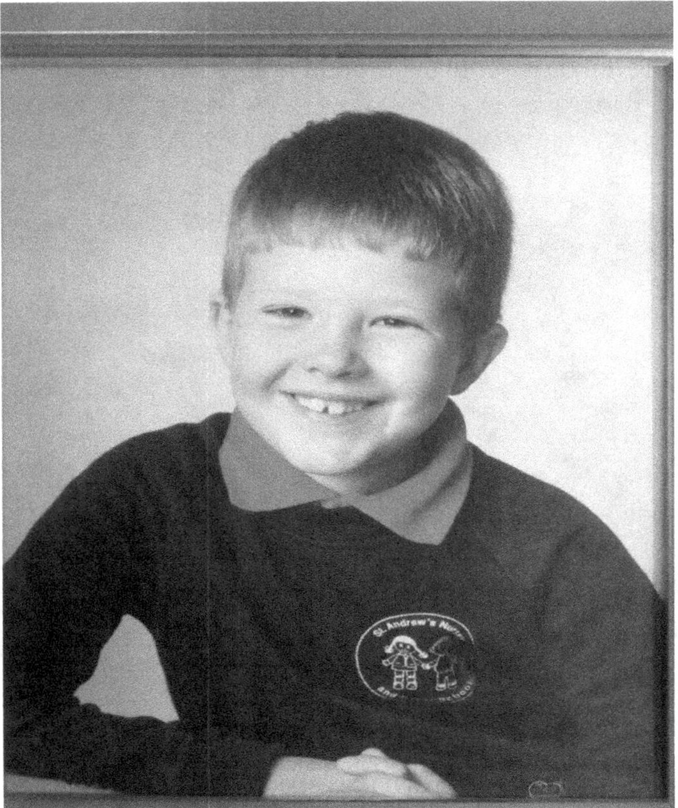
Lloyd wearing his school uniform.

After nursery school came the reception class.

Schools liked Mum's helping, but not to be there constantly, not like they did in the nursery. But I got around this by becoming a dinner lady in Lloyd's class. And this way, I could be around him at lunchtime.

I also helped a lot in his class, and Lloyd was so proud because I was his dinner lady.

He was a very fit, energetic little lad. Well, not so little, because Lloyd was tall for his age and towered over his class friends and many pupils in the older classes.

Lloyd never suffered from any common illnesses, and I have never had too many myself.

Lloyd had a special friend in his life, and they were like twins.

They even looked very much alike when you saw them together, and always had such brilliant fun with each other.

You would think they were brothers, very fond of each other and always spending lots of time together. Lloyd had a lot of fun, and we went on many caravanning holidays. Touring around is splendid fun.

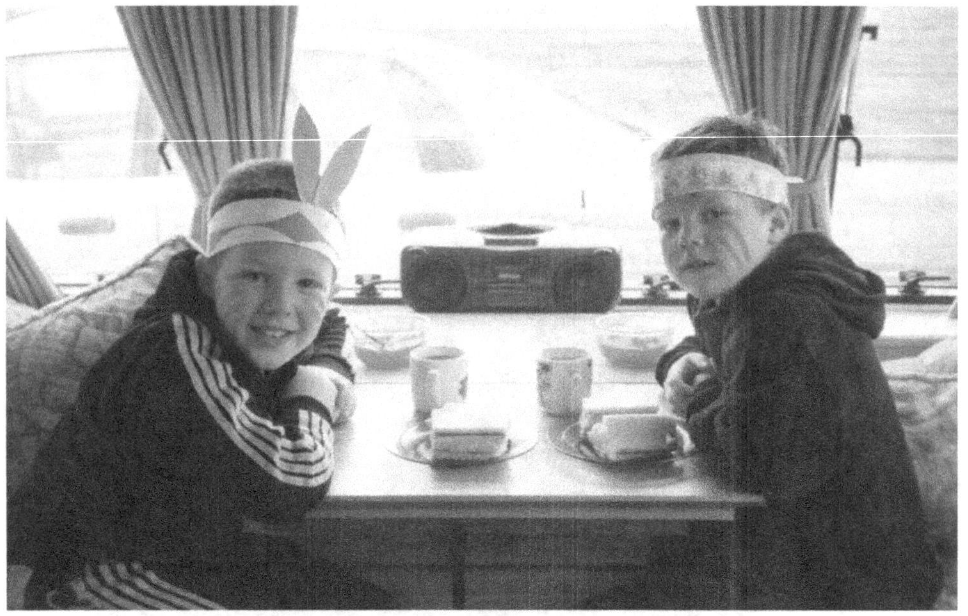

Lloyd and and his best friend, Adam, in our caravan in Devon.

Lloyd loved school and always had respect for his teachers and elders. He enjoyed sports days and would compete in and win lots of races.

Mind you, Lloyd's legs were long, and before I knew it, Lloyd was in year one and best mates with Adam, enjoying life to the full, and I was still his dinner lady.

And when Lloyd went up a year, I also changed classes until Lloyd began Junior school.

When leaving the infants' school, I worked in the Royal Gwent Hospital. It upset Lloyd to see me go, but the hours were long, and higher wages came with the job.

The best thing about it was that I could take Lloyd to school, which I loved. I would watch him queue up in his line with his backpack, towering over everyone else, and we would wave goodbye to each other when he was going into his class.

Although he was older, we still had that special bond. And always emotional with each other.

I was often home from work on time for Lloyd because my job had the same working hours as Lloyd's school times, so we got used to it. But we still missed each other during the dinner hour break.

So, on my day off from work during the week, we would visit the local park for a picnic. I also helped the teachers on their school trips.

Lloyd found it hard when his special friend, Adam, moved away.

Adam was no longer with Lloyd during the week or at school. During this time, I could sense Lloyd's loneliness, and we grew even closer to each other.

I played with Lloyd a lot when Adam was there, but since Adam left, we have become extra-special friends and do everything together.

He didn't want to play with other children, and it was always me he wanted. And this was my role as a mum, to be Lloyd's soul mate. We idolised each other.

I then took Lloyd to Cub Scouts, where I helped, and he also began Judo lessons.

Lloyd loved swimming; he was a fantastic swimmer.

He worked hard in the pool, and his determination earned him a gold certificate. Lloyd taught me to swim.

We went swimming a lot together.

Lloyd also taught me about caring. He was always loving towards everyone he met.

Such a beautiful little soul.

Chapter Two.

Shattered Dreams.

Little before Lloyd left Infant's school to go up to Juniors, he had an eye test. The school nurse referred Lloyd to the opticians for a thorough eye examination.

Lloyd was seven years old. We went to the opticians, and they gave Lloyd a pair of glasses, which made him feel 'cool' when he wore them.

We paid for a special glasses case for them. Lloyd and I thought they suited him, and he looked handsome when he wore them.

He only needed to wear glasses for reading and watching TV. As the months passed, Lloyd's teacher and I noticed the spectacles weren't helping as they should, so we returned to the opticians.

This time, we spoke to somebody different. Upon examination, Lloyd's eyes raised concerns about his left eye, so they advised me to take Lloyd to our doctor.

So, we went to our doctor and explained the optician's findings, and he referred us to the Ophthalmology Department at the Royal Gwent Hospital.

For the time being, Lloyd continued wearing his glasses for reading. Soon after, we received a letter with an appointment to attend the Ophthalmology Unit on 21 November 1998.

Lloyd was tested and found to have a slight hypermetropic (long-sighted) refractive error. They reviewed Lloyd at St. Woolos Hospital in Wales on 24 February 1999.

The result of the review was poor vision in the right eye.

His visual acuity (vision sharpness) was to be 6/18 unaided in the right eye and 6/36 in the left eye (i.e., worse in the left eye).

The orthoptist found improved vision when she pointed to the letters, and then Lloyd achieved 6/6 unaided in the right eye (normal vision) and 6/9 in the left eye.

They recommended occlusion therapy (patching the expert eye to encourage the use of the critical eye), so Lloyd had to wear an eye patch for three months.

They removed the eye patch just in time for our holiday of a lifetime to Disney

World, Florida. I always promised we would go sometime.

It is a magical kingdom for all ages.

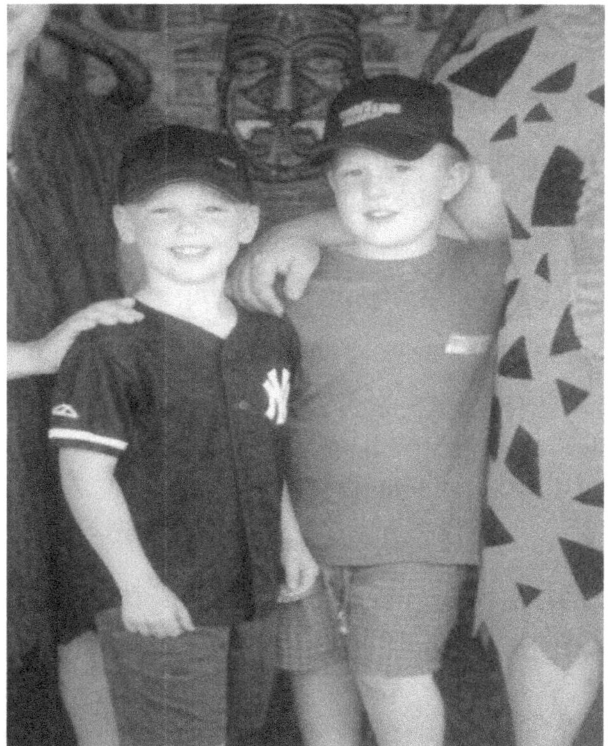

Lloyd and his best friend, Adam, with the Flintstones in Florida.

Our hotel was splendid, and the water parks were fun, so Lloyd and his special friend Adam loved every minute of our fortnight's holiday.

We have many photos and videos to remember our fabulous time in Florida. I also have pictures and videos of us since Lloyd was born.

Having kept his first shoes, pieces of hair, and everything he possessed through the years, I will always keep them. I feel I need to.

As the months progressed, I noticed a change in Lloyd. In Florida, he seemed weak, tired, and was coming home from school, worn out for a child his age.

I also noticed Lloyd was bumping into things.

When he walked through the doors, he would walk into the door frames. And when watching the TV, his head was tilted to one side as if he was looking through one eye.

Another thing I noticed was that Lloyd was drinking a lot of water, so I took him to the doctor for a diabetes check.

Lloyd was fine. But all these months of noticing the changes bothered me. He couldn't play ball games in Cub Scouts because he didn't know where the ball was coming from. He could not see it.

His Judo lessons were proving harder because he was so weak.

One day, Lloyd told me he had a headache at school. A friend, a dinner lady in Lloyd's school, said he hadn't been playing as usual at playtime.

He would sit in the corner of the play yard on his own. I felt so hurt that my bubbly, happy little boy was upset and not feeling well.

I would not take no for an answer, and needed to sort this out.

So in October 1999, five months later, I contacted the Ophthalmology department in St. Woolos Hospital and explained that Lloyd was bumping into things and having difficulty looking from one thing to another.

They made an appointment for 13 October 1999.

Lloyd's visual acuity remained unchanged, and they further assessed it. Examination of the Fundus (the part of the eye behind the pupil) showed no abnormality.

They felt no further investigation or treatment was necessary, so Lloyd was discharged from the clinic.

I was furious because I felt something was wrong with my Lloyd. So I started from the beginning, but this time to see a different specialist.

I returned with Lloyd to the opticians, where we purchased his glasses, and asked if we could see a different optician.

The other optician could not improve Lloyd's vision with fresher glasses, but noted he was bumping into things.

He also found that both optic discs (where nerve fibres from the retina leave the eye) were pale.

So they reviewed Lloyd in the Orthoptic Clinic on 7 April 2000. They measured his visual acuity as 6/18 in the right eye, improving to 6/9 with encouragement. And 6/24 in the left eye.

The Orthoptist felt that they should examine Lloyd at the Consultant Ophthalmic clinic, so they arranged an appointment for Lloyd on 11 July 2000.

They cancelled this because the doctor was unwell, and offered no further appointment as they didn't know when the doctor would return to work.

I needed to do something as soon as possible. So, instead of waiting. On 23 June 2000, I arranged for a private doctor to test Lloyd's vision for 75 pounds.

I wish we had seen this doctor from the start.

After his examination, the doctor found Lloyd's visual acuity was 6/24 in the right eye and 6/60 in the left eye, and there was no improvement with additional lenses.

His colour vision was poor, both optic discs were pale, and he couldn't see things on his right-hand side.

It concerned the doctor that there may be an underlying neurological problem, so he arranged for Lloyd to have an MRI brain scan.

They scheduled the scan for 17 July 2000.

Well. I don't know why. But from the day the doctor mentioned that Lloyd needed an MRI scan, for some unknown reason, something was telling me Lloyd had a brain tumour.

It had shattered our lives.

People told me to wait until the scan results, but I knew, call it a mother's instinct.

Oh, please, God, don't let my precious child have a brain tumour. I kept praying over and over. Please, God, no, not my Lloyd.

17 July 2000 was approaching, and I needed to prepare Lloyd for his scan because an MRI scanner can be daunting for a child.

I knew what the scanner looked like because I worked at the Royal Gwent Hospital, where Lloyd's scan would happen, and I had seen this machine.

I needed strength to help my little angel through his journey of courage. So, I told Lloyd about his upcoming MRI scan and drew a picture of the machine.

I told him to pretend it was a rocket ship lying down, and he is an astronaut. Then, you will sit at the foot of the spaceship. They will lay you down, secure your head so you can't move it, and they will slowly put you into your rocket.

When you hear a loud noise, it's the equipment. Don't worry, my darling, pretend the rocket is taking off, so close your eyes and imagine you can see the stars.

17 July 2000 arrived. And Lloyd was a brave astronaut, but unbeknownst to me, Lloyd needed an injection to add dye to his bloodstream.

I explained this to him as best I could, and he said, " That's fine. He's so brave.

It stung him going in. Lloyd said he could feel the cold dye flowing through his veins. But he never complained. He just explained how it felt.

It upset me because I hadn't told him about everything that would happen and hadn't prepared him for the injection.

While Lloyd was inside the scanning machine, I stayed with him, holding his foot and leg so he could feel I was with him.

It seemed like a long time since he was in the scanner, and it was also very noisy.

When he came out, I praised him and told him how brave he was. He said, "That wasn't too terrible, mum." And so, from then on, I called him my brave little soldier.

After the scan, we went to Newport Town so I could treat him to something. He deserved it because of his bravery.

Lloyd wasn't a stranger to pain. When he was five years old, he had to have an anaesthetic to put him to sleep, as he needed a front tooth removed. He had an abscess behind the tooth root, and the dentist decided he should remove it.

The dentist said Lloyd could feel groggy after the procedure. But when he came round, he was running around the surgery as if he had nothing done to him.

When they put Lloyd under anaesthetic, it upset and worried me about him going to sleep. But he was fine.

They invited Lloyd to his friend's birthday party, where they had a bouncy castle.

He loved bouncy castles and was having a glorious time. And when he bounced off and onto the padded mats, he cried, saying his shoulder was hurting him.

Later, we saw his shoulder didn't look right, so we took him to the casualty department at the Royal Gwent Hospital.

The doctors discovered he had broken his collarbone, so they put his arm in a sling. Lloyd is as brave as usual. He never moaned once and said he felt 'cool' with his arm in a sling.

On another occasion, a few months before he began visiting the opticians about his eyes, he was playing with a friend.

Lloyd was pulling the living room door open, and his friend was on the other side, pulling it shut. His friend let go of the door, but Lloyd was pulling it with such force that the door went over Lloyd's big toe.

It lifted his toenail and split it. He began screaming in pain, so I had to take him to the casualty department.

They said his nail required removal, but didn't want to put Lloyd to sleep, so they injected his toe in several places with a local anaesthetic.

Now. Lloyd could see everything the doctors were doing, and when they used a pair of pliers, he panicked.

He shouted out as the doctors pulled and tugged at his nail. I felt awful to see him going through that, but after they bandaged his toe, Lloyd settled down a little. And when they mentioned crutches, it impressed him.

When we went home, he waited at our front door for his school friends to come down the street so he could show them his bandaged toe and his crutches.

The doctor who treated Lloyd said that he would feel a lot of pain in his toe, but as usual, Lloyd, being Lloyd, never complained.

After Lloyd had his MRI scan on 17 July 2000, I had a terrible feeling there would be some tumour because of his symptoms and the fact that he needed a scan. I am terrified.

I received a letter from the hospital, informing me that the doctor I had paid wanted to see Lloyd and me at the Optical Department in St. Woolos Hospital on 20 July 2000.

My heart missed a beat because results like this take a long time, and I received this letter only three days after the MRI scan.

It worried me because I knew deep in my heart that these results would be devastating.

The 20th day of July came, and my deepest worries are proving correct.

They sat us in the office with the doctor and one of his colleagues. They put an X-ray on a lighted screen and explained to Lloyd that they had found a lump in his head and would tell him about it as best they could.

I knew Lloyd was a very sensible boy for his age, and he deserved to know about the lump and that he would understand.

The doctor continued by saying that the MRI scan showed the lump in Lloyd's head was a tumour, and they'd do everything to help him and put it right.

Lloyd said, "Okay, doctor, that's fine, thank you."

The nurse in the office took Lloyd out of the room for a short while to show him some equipment they used to test people's eyes, so that the doctor could have a private word with me.

He told me the tumour was large and in his left optic tract. The optic tract? It forms part of the nervous system, and these fibres carry information from the eyes to the brain.

It stunned me. My words were, "Why has this happened? He's only a child. Why? How did it get there? Please help him and remove this tumour."

Please, this can't be happening to us. What have we ever done to deserve this?

As you can understand, it upset me. Then Lloyd returned to the office as happy as ever and told me what the nurse had shown him.

The doctor said to Lloyd. "Lloyd, we will plan for you to go into the hospital for some tests, and it will be the University Hospital of Wales in Cardiff."

Lloyd replied. "Okay, doctor. I don't mind."

He is so understanding.

I don't know what came over me. I ran out of the doctor's office, past the reception area, and out to the front of the hospital, where I began screaming and crying.

The nurse came outside to me with Lloyd, and he put his arms around me and said, "Don't cry, mum. I'll be fine. It's only a lump, and they can take it away? I don't like to see you cry, Mum. I've never seen you cry before. And I don't want to see you cry again, mum. Please don't."

I felt so ashamed, crying like that in front of Lloyd, and I said to him, "Lloyd, I am so very sorry for crying. It's just that mummy's sad because you are going to the hospital. I promise I will never cry again."

We hugged each other.

The same morning, I decided that I would no longer work because I needed to be with my boy, and I didn't think Lloyd would have to go to school again because of what he needed to have done.

So, Lloyd and I went to the Royal Gwent Hospital, where I worked, and told my manager about what was happening. She understood and said. "When you are ready, there will always be a job here for you."

She's wonderful.

I had such a sad feeling inside me, but I needed to put on a brave face for Lloyd, so I took him to the town, bought him a present, and then went to his favourite McDonald's for a burger.

And this was the day I realised that my wonderful life with my gorgeous little child would change. So I needed all my strength for Lloyd and not to leave his side.

We have always been very close, but now I knew I would never leave his side.

A few days after the MRI scan results, I received a letter telling me to go to the University Hospital of Wales for Lloyd to get admitted.

We went to the South Paediatric Ward and settled ourselves. On our first day there, we saw many doctors.

The doctors wanted to see me in private, so the nurse played with Lloyd. He needed to have blood taken for testing, along with urine samples.

They asked many questions about our background, mostly about other family members who may have similar problems, for instance, cancer and brain tumours.

I explained that my mother died of cancer, and my father died of a heart problem. There were so many questions to answer.

It was awful to see Lloyd having another needle because they hurt, even though this time, the doctors were using a cream known as Ametop to deaden the area.

They were having trouble finding Lloyd's vein, so they looked for another one and couldn't get blood there either. At last, after trying four times, they obtained the blood for testing.

The doctors told me they were sorry Lloyd's veins were difficult to find.

Lloyd needed to see a doctor who would explain what would happen. We were to stay in the hospital for a few days while having tests, then go home for a little while, and return on 3 August 2000 for an operation.

There are two things they have to do during the operation. One was a biopsy. They needed this to find out more about the tumour. And the second was to fit a shunt.

He needs a shunt because there's a lot of fluid in Lloyd's head, and this makes him feel giddy. The shunt will drain the fluid from his head into his stomach and disappear, so that he wouldn't feel giddy any more.

A shunt is a small device fitted just behind his ear. It has a tube which goes down the inside of the neck and travels down the body into the stomach.

The doctor explained that he would cut Lloyd's head, one on his tummy and another on top of his head, for the biopsy.

They reassured Lloyd that it wouldn't hurt because he would be fast asleep, and then he explained the anaesthetic.

Lloyd said. "Okay, doctor, thank you. I'll be fine. See you on 3 August 2000."S

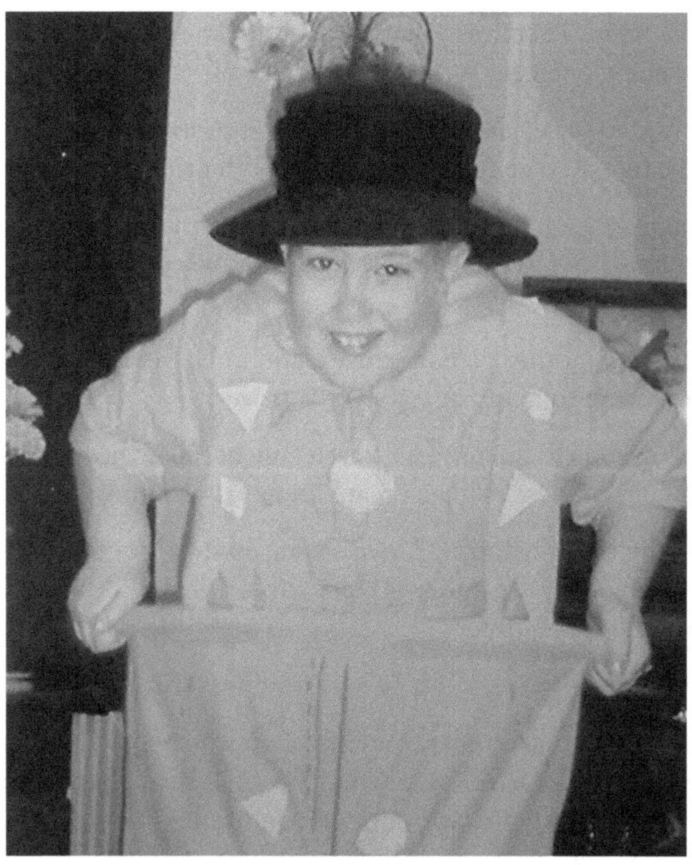

Chapter Three.

Make Life Special.

So, I decided, from that day on, that I would make Lloyd's life enjoyable and exceptional and not worry about money.

Money means nothing any more, and I will spend everything on whatever it takes to make Lloyd happy before we need to go back to the hospital on 3 August.

I wanted to take Lloyd to Pontins for some fun. So I planned to go there for a week with my friend Shirley and her daughter, Paige.

We arrived at Pontin's holiday park, and Lloyd thought it was great. He loved the water, so we went swimming, and he enjoyed going to the arcades. They were fantastic.

And he also loved the two-pence drop machine and the electric quad bikes.

I made every moment as happy as I could. But my heart was in pieces thinking of how much this wonderful child would go through and wishing I could take his place.

So I had to put a brave face on all the time, which is difficult when all your dreams have come to an end. But I need to make the rest of our time together extra special.

As we continue through the book, I will explain about our happy moments together and the sad ones.

One day on our holiday, Lloyd went on a go-kart. So I put a helmet on his head, strapped him in, and then he had to go around a track.

He was going around, having fun, until a man put up a flag to stop. And because of his poor eyesight, Lloyd crashed into the back of another lad who had stopped.

I shouted, "Oh my God! " and ran straight over to Lloyd, removing his helmet to check his head. Thank God he was okay, but it shook us both up.

Later that evening, when Lloyd and my friend's daughter were sleeping, I spoke to Shirley and said. "I am terrified they won't be able to remove the tumour."

Shirley, a sympathetic friend, replied. "Yes, they will. Lloyd will be fine, don't worry."

But it's impossible not to worry.

Anyway. We were on holiday, and I had to make it extra special.

The next day, we visited a shop and bought some lovely presents for Lloyd. I needed him to have anything he wanted, and I would say. "You are a special boy, and I want to buy you gifts."

Lloyd said. "Is it because I have a brain tumour, mum?"

I replied. "No, darling. You have always been special to me, and I want to buy you gifts because I love you."

Lloyd said. "I love you too, mum. You are special to me, too."

The following morning, Lloyd kissed me and said. "Good morning, mum."

I felt like a princess kissed by a prince. So I told Lloyd, and he thought it was a sweet thing to say.

We had to leave for home that day, ready to go to the hospital. I haven't been able to get the 3rd day of August out of my mind, and the thought of my baby going through all that pain. But I am Lloyd's mother, nurse and best friend, and I will never leave his side. We have a powerful bond and special love for each other.

It's the 3rd day of August 2000, and our first day in the U.H.W. Cardiff Paediatrics Ward South, but we are not in a shared ward.

We have a room of our own and have settled in. The nursing staff are fantastic, and Lloyd is fine. As he always says, "I'm fine."

The doctor wanted to talk with me in private, so a nurse stayed in our room and played with Lloyd.

The neurosurgeon, a brilliant man, explained what they would do, including the potential problems.

For example, he informed me about the dangers of operating on the head and why it's required. It is to diagnose the tumour and determine whether it is benign or malignant.

He also told me that when they fit the shunt, Lloyd can't play any contact sports such as football, rugby, or judo.

Lloyd's not bothered about football or rugby, but he loves judo. And this made me feel sad for him.

But I know my Lloyd, he will understand.

The neurosurgeon told me Lloyd has to go to a High Dependency ward after his operation for twenty-four hours. And this bothered me because I know how dangerous operating on the head is.

The anaesthetist came into the room where the surgeon and I were conversing to explain his requirements. And then we left the room and went to see Lloyd.

Lloyd thought the anaesthetist was great.

He said. "Lloyd, I will give you a bit of gas to make you sleepy. And then I will insert some anaesthetic into your body so you will stay asleep through your operation, and you won't even know you have had it done."

Lloyd replied. "That's fine."

He wasn't at all frightened.

Lloyd hadn't been able to eat or drink for hours, which was awful for him. He loves his food and drink. I wouldn't eat or drink until he could.

I explained to Lloyd that he could no longer play any contact sport, and he said, "I don't mind for now, as long as I get better."

By now, I am so worried. Lots of awful things go through your mind.

At one stage, I thought if the worst thing happened to Lloyd, I'd go with him. I couldn't stand the thought of life without my Lloyd.

When they came for Lloyd, I stayed with him while they gave him the anaesthetic. And this is such an emotional experience when they put your baby to sleep for a life-threatening operation.

I held his hand, kissed him, and said. "Sweet dreams, Lloyd. Mummy loves you." They then asked me to leave the room.

Lloyd was in the theatre for five hours. And it was the worst five hours of my life, and for everyone else who knew him.

After five hours, I received a call from the nurse, who told me Lloyd was out of the theatre and in recovery. My feet didn't touch the ground, and I was like a bolt of lightning heading to the recovery room.

And when I went in, his eyes were open, and I thanked God. I kissed Lloyd and said, "I love you, darling."

Then I asked him if he was alright, and guess what he said? "I'm fine." And this is his favourite saying.

But he wasn't. He needed to go to the High Dependency Ward because his blood pressure was sky-high, through the roof, and he had lost the use of his right arm and leg.

So, they tested him for arm and leg movement because of the biopsy.

The left side of the brain (where his tumour is) tells the right side of your body what to do, and vice versa. His oxygen level was low, and his pulse wasn't right, so he was sent to High Dependency.

When we were there, they put Lloyd on a heart monitor, pulse machine, and blood pressure machine, and he was taking in oxygen from a mask over his mouth.

He wasn't talking, and his eyes were closed. I didn't leave him at all. I couldn't. I needed to assist Lloyd, doing whatever I could to help him.

As the hours passed, they decided Lloyd needed a catheter to help him pass urine. He hadn't had a pee for a long while and also needed fluids via a drip.

I was angry about him having a catheter because it should've been fitted during the operation while Lloyd was under anaesthetic.

I explained to him that the doctors would fit a tube in his penis to help him pass urine, so he wouldn't have to keep getting up to go to the toilet (he couldn't anyway), and it would go down the tube into a plastic bag.

So when he needed to go to the toilet, he didn't have to worry.

It was disgusting how they pushed the tube through Lloyd's penis. He screamed out in pain. I felt like hitting the nurse and seeing how he would like it if I were to push the catheter into his penis.

You get angry seeing your child in so much pain. I know the nurse is only doing what is for the best. They're wonderful. But it is still very upsetting.

I hugged Lloyd and settled him down, and then the neurosurgeon came to see me and said Lloyd needed an X-ray on his head to find out what was causing his arm and leg problems.

He needed to go to the X-ray department, but I wasn't happy about moving him. But we had to, so we wheeled Lloyd down in his bed.

When we arrived at the X-ray department, they moved Lloyd onto the X-ray bed and placed his head between two wedges to stop him from moving his head.

Lloyd gave out a scream, and this was because the wedges of the X-ray machine were pressing on the cut where he had his biopsy and where they had fitted the shunt. He also had staples in his head, and I thought to myself, I can't let him go through any more. I was getting annoyed, but they explained the reason for this.

Well, what can you do? It is important.

Lloyd calmed down, so I hugged him and said. "I will call you Brave Heart because I have known no one as brave as you."

The nurses agreed and gave him some stickers for bravery. They took us back to the High Dependency Department, and we waited for the X-ray results.

When the results came back, they showed Lloyd's loss of movement with his arm and leg was due to swelling caused by the surgery from the biopsy.

The swelling had contacted the nerve endings and caused the problems, so they needed to put Lloyd on steroids to control the swelling. We know the steroids as Hydrocortisone.

Lloyd also has very high blood pressure and needs to take blood pressure tablets known as Nifedipine, which will help him while he is on a blood pressure machine to keep it under control.

They have allowed us to return to our ward, so we feel a little more settled in our room. Lloyd is sleeping all the time and is weak. I feel so emotional, but I need to keep strong and smile, which is tough.

Remember, I promised Lloyd that he would never see me cry again. So I will keep a smile on my face for him. Try to keep things as normal as possible for your child's sake because your feelings cannot get in the way. And no matter what, you must give them 100% care and attention.

The anaesthetic has worn off, and Lloyd is in considerable pain, so they have given him powerful pain relief. Lloyd cannot sit up yet because of the swelling in his head, so they move his head from side to side. It's breaking my heart to see my baby boy like this.

He has been lying flat for several days. It is now 7 August, and there has been no change. This afternoon, I have to meet the surgeon to get the results of Lloyd's biopsy. I'm unsure whether it's a mother's instinct, and I don't enjoy feeling this way, but I fear it will be grave news.

Just looking at the way he is now after a biopsy, I don't think they will be able to remove the tumour.

Chapter Four.

Why Is This Happening To Us?

My meeting with Mr Hatfield and his colleague was what I'd expected.

They said, "We are very sorry to give you this sad news, but Lloyd's brain tumour is malignant and inoperable because it is a rare tumour, very invasive and close to the brain stem. Lloyd needs treatment as soon as possible because of the growing speed of the tumour, or he will only live for another three months. So we will use chemotherapy treatment, to begin with, followed by radiotherapy."

It shattered my world; I'm speechless.

Why is this happening to us?

What have we ever done to deserve it?

Can I keep myself strong enough to get through this?

Yes, I must, and I promise I'll be there every step of the way to guide him through it and keep things as normal as possible.

Please, God, help us get through this.

It is now 9 August, and I will explain things to him when we return home, and he's feeling better.

I will try to explain the best I can without frightening him.

Today, I have sat Lloyd up, and he has opened his eyes a little, so I moved the headrest. But as soon as we lifted Lloyd a small way, he said he felt sick and could see nothing.

He said everything went black.

The doctor came to see him and told us it was due to the pressure in his head, and he would be alright. Then after a short while, Lloyd's vision returned, and he felt better, so he sat up further. It was great to see him smile again; He has such a gorgeous smile.

I stayed with him all the time and slept by his side because I couldn't be away from him for five minutes and needed to be with him.

Lloyd had his catheter removed today, and it hurt, but not as badly as the insertion. He can sit up this morning and will use a urine bottle.

Tomorrow, they want Lloyd to get up because the physiotherapy nurses are coming to help him walk a few steps.

The doctor says he needs to do this as soon as possible.

It's 10 August, and we helped Lloyd out of bed, but he felt unwell, so they are leaving him in his wheelchair for a while.

We'll wait outside our room until the nurses return and try again.

Two hours later, the nurses returned, and we got Lloyd out of his wheelchair and walked him down the hospital corridor and back.

He did well, and the nurse was pleased; he is also trying to use his arm, and it's coming along nicely.

This afternoon, Lloyd's having the staples removed from his head and tummy, so they are giving him extra pain relief to help with this.

I was so worried about him having the staples removed, and as usual, Lloyd said, "I don't mind, and please can I keep them, and please don't worry, I will be fine."

The nurses are preparing to remove the staples, and I hold Lloyd's hand because they will use surgical grippers to remove them.

When removing the staples, I could feel everyone coming out, but Lloyd never moaned once and said, "Is that it? Are they all out now?"

The nurses put all the removed staples in a pot for Lloyd to keep.

Lloyd is a brave little soldier, and I love him very much.

We now know his wheelchair as Lloyd's Chariot, and he doesn't mind being in it, and he's now getting used to it.

This afternoon, they are taking Lloyd off his blood pressure machine, as the Nifedipine blood pressure tablets don't seem to control his blood pressure as the doctors had hoped. But he needs to keep taking them until further notice.

Later, we are going down to the shops, in the hospital concourse, to treat Lloyd to a deserved gift.

It will probably be a teddy or two as he collects teddy bears and has hundreds of them.

So off we go in his chariot.

The sad thing about going to the shops was that everyone was looking at the back of Lloyd's head.

It was all shaved with two massive scars and a lump where they fitted the shunt, but we're happy to get around because the operation could have been fatal. But thank God Lloyd got through it; he is such a Braveheart.

We bought many lovely things for him, and at one time, Lloyd put on a pair of headphones and listened to music.

While in the shop, I noticed a blue card on a stand that caught my eye.

I picked it up, and when I read it, my eyes filled with tears. But I had to be careful that Lloyd didn't see me because I felt the words of this poem were for me.

And I believe they meant for me to find and purchase this poem, so I did, and this is what it said.

God's Lent Child.

I'll lend you a little while, a child of mine. God said.

For you to love them while he lives and mourn for them when he's dead?

It may be six or seven years or forty-two or three.

But will you, till I call him back, take care of him for me?

He'll bring his charms to gladden you,

And should his stay be brief?

You'll always have his memories,

As a solace for your grief.

I cannot promise he will stay,

Since all from earth returns.

But there are lessons taught below,

That I want this child to learn.

I've looked the entire world over,

In search of teachers, true,

And from the things that crowd life's lane,

I have chosen you.

Now, will you give him all your love?

Nor think the labour vain,

Or hate me when I come to take this lent child back again?

I fancied I heard them say,

Dear Lord, thy will is done,

For all the joys thy child will bring,

The risk of grief we'll run.

We'll shelter him with tenderness,

We'll love him while we may,

And for the happiness we've known forever, more grateful we stay.

But should those angels call for him?

Much sooner than we planned,

We'll brave the bitter grief that comes.

And try to understand.

We returned to our room, and the doctor was there waiting; he checked Lloyd and said, "We will let you go home tomorrow, young man, but only if you promise to rest."

Lloyd replied, "I promise I will rest."

I'm pleased we can return home because I want to make things very special for Lloyd.

It thrills Lloyd that we can take his chariot home with us.

We were leaving for home the following day, and we couldn't wait, so we said goodbye to the hospital staff, who were fabulous people; Lloyd loved them.

When we returned home, we found the house windows covered in balloons and a banner that read, Welcome Home, Lloydy: It thrilled us.

We went into the house, but Lloyd needed to lie down and sleep for a few hours as he gets more tired by the day.

The next day, I found out that there's a fun day planned for Lloyd at our local public house, The Star Inn, to welcome him home.

An excellent friend of ours, Yvonne, with other friends, had got together and planned the day.

They are all special people to us, and Lloyd loved them; they all loved him very much.

When Lloyd woke up after resting, I told him about the planned fun day and asked if he would like to go. But only if he felt well enough, and because Lloyd has a lot of sense for an adolescent boy, he replied, "I will go if I feel okay."

That afternoon, we played some of his games, and it was fabulous being together and spending such precious moments.

We played draughts, snakes and ladders, dominoes and a card game called "UNO", which Lloyd enjoyed playing, and we went to bed early, looking forward to the next day because it was Lloyd's Fun Day.

And it's going to be a busy day?

The following morning, Lloyd woke and said, "I would love to go to my fun day, Mum."

So, later that morning, we went to The Star Inn, and what a day that was because there were lots of things for the children to do and a barbecue.

All the men wore white t-shirts with fun names they had made up for themselves printed on the front.

They made one for Lloyd, which read in big red letters: LLOYD PIKE THE PINT.

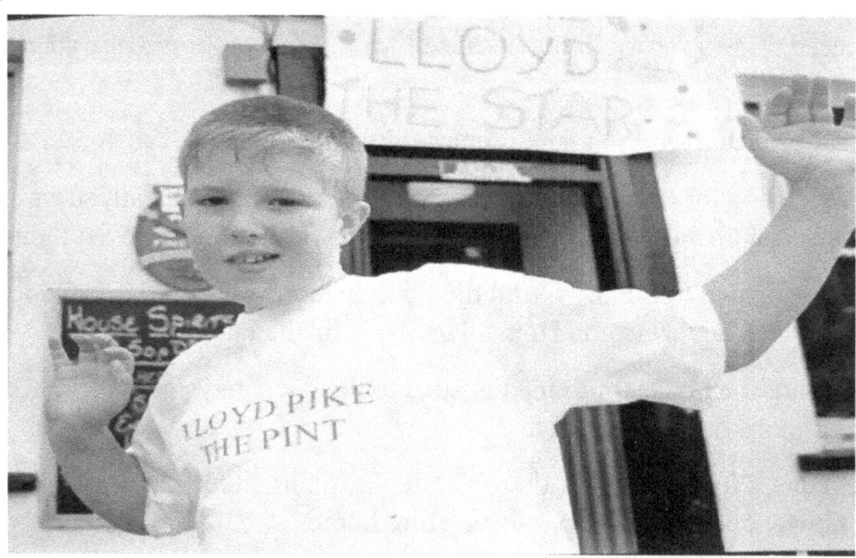

Lloyd thought it was great because they even had funny wigs and were in fancy dress, and many friends of ours came from everywhere, near and far; all went to plan, and Lloyd had lots of fun.

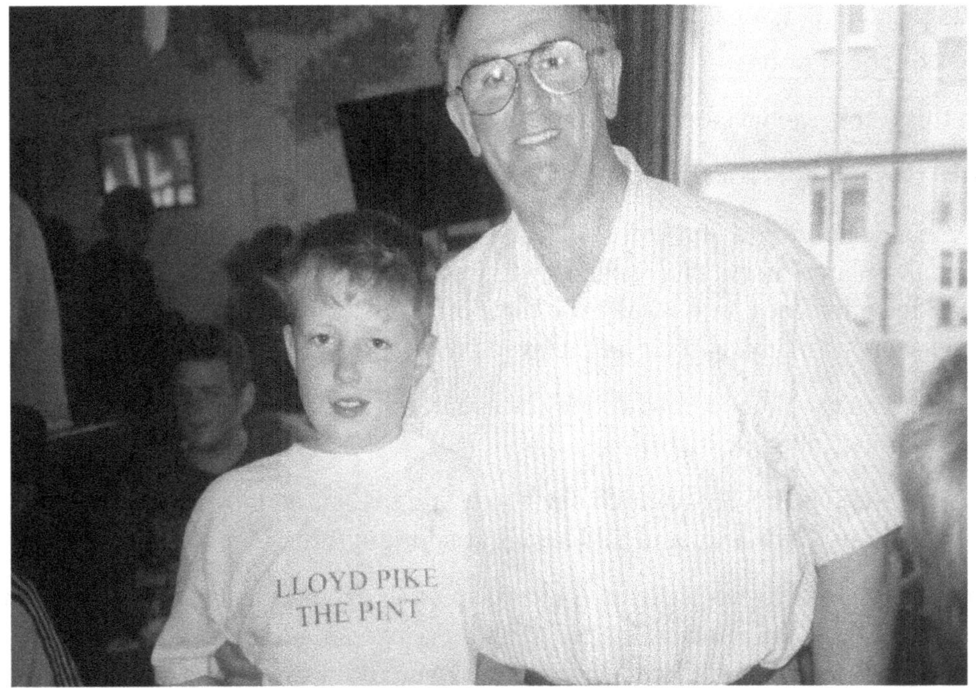

Lloyd with his Grandpa John.

I kept asking him if he was alright, and as usual, he replied, "I'm fine."

So I replied, " Please tell me when you are ready to go home."

Later, after a fantastic time with all our friends and family, which exhausted Lloyd, we returned home.

The next day, in the afternoon, and after Lloyd had had his usual two hours of sleep, they asked us to return to The Star Inn.

When we arrived, the pub was full of friends and family, and they asked Lloyd to sit in the lounge in the middle of the room.

They gave him a get-well card, and when he opened it, lots of money fell out. Lloyd's face was a picture, and our friend Yvonne told Lloyd to throw it in the air.

We filmed the fun day and also took loads of photographs.

Videos and photos are a must-do for memories with your child, whether they are ill or not.

Our family and friends raised the money in the card from the fun day for Lloyd to spend on whatever he wanted.

Lloyd had everything he wanted, so we took him to lovely places because he loved fairgrounds and arcades and used to enjoy fast rides, but now he only goes on the slow ones.

So this week, we have been busy visiting some brilliant places.

Next week, they are having another event for Lloyd in a club.

My wonderful friend Hayley, who is organising it, will shave her brother's hair. He has a plait which he has been growing since he was a young boy. The plait goes down his back, and when they cut it off, they'll auction it. Other friends of Hayley are also having their hair shaved off.

Lloyd wasn't well enough to attend the event, but they gave us many photos; it was another fantastic night.

Hayley and her brother came to our house and presented Lloyd with the money they had raised for him, and told him it was for anything that pleased him.

People's generosity overwhelmed Lloyd, and he's grateful to everybody for what they have done for him and for planning these events. I am also so grateful to these people, some of whom never knew Lloyd, and these events helped us have many enjoyable and memorable times together and to take Lloyd wherever he wanted.

It is Monday, 14 August, and we have bought a dog, a King Charles Spaniel.

We went to a lady's house who was a dog breeder. And as you can imagine, she had quite a few puppies running around. But one puppy in particular ran straight to Lloyd and began jumping upon him, so we told the lady that this was the one we wanted.

He is gorgeous, and we immediately named him Lucky because he was lucky to have Lloyd. Lloyd loves him very much. They fell asleep on the settee together, so I took a photograph of them.

It's beautiful.

Chapter Five.

Please, God, help us through our journey.

Lloyd hasn't been feeling very well this week because he sleeps a lot, is weak, and due to the steroids, he is eating a lot, but I am not worried about it.

He feels uncomfortable and is sweating profusely; he is sweating buckets.

Lloyds specialist will now wean him off the steroids, and the swelling in his head is also going down.

But when I was weaning Lloyd off his steroids, he began having severe headaches, so I contacted the specialist, who kept Lloyd on them until further notice.

As the days and weeks passed, it upset me that back in 1998, when I first took Lloyd to the hospital about his eyes, they said all he had was a lazy eye.

So they patched it for three months and said we no longer needed to see Lloyd; this was three months wasted?

So I paid a private doctor, Doctor Blythe, who used the same equipment in his surgery as in the Orthoptic Department, and Doctor Blythe found the grey vessels behind the eye.

So why didn't the St. Woolos Orthoptic Department find the grey vessels behind Lloyd's eye?

I wrote a letter of complaint to St. Woolos, saying I believed if they had picked up the grey vessels in 1998, perhaps the tumour wouldn't have grown so much during those wasted three months.

There was no reply to my complaint, and I wish I had paid privately and seen Doctor Blythe earlier.

Tuesday, 22 August, Lloyd is still sleepy and needs his wheelchair because of his weakness.

Today, a specialist nurse is coming to the house to speak with Lloyd about having a device fitted into his chest so they can insert a needle into it to make it easier for Lloyd.

The nurse's name is Rachel, and she has a doll with a device fitted to it; this makes it easier when explaining it to a child.

They know the device as a Port-a-Cath. And she said they fit it while you are asleep in the hospital, just like when you had the other operation.

You won't feel anything, and the doctor will make a cut in your chest and another minor cut on the side of your neck.

And then they will install a plug-type fitment, with a sponge in the middle, into your chest that has a tube going under your skin, up to your neck and then into the jugular vein.

So when we put a needle into the port, we can draw blood out, and we can also use it to give you chemotherapy treatment.

Many children either have a port or a Hickman line.

The difference is that a port is under your skin, so you can still go swimming, but a Hickman line has tubes hanging on the outside, so swimming is a big no-no.

Lloyd will have the port device fitted on 5 September (partner's birthday) and a lumbar puncture, a needle in the spine for testing for certain uncommon ailments.

Then, the following morning, they would like to start Lloyd on his chemotherapy treatment, one of which is carboplatin, the other being vincristine.

Before 5 September, they need to conduct a kidney function test. And they will take blood every hour for four hours; this will take place on 24 August.

Thursday, 24 August. Llandough Hospital, Penarth, Oncology Ward.

Everyone is fantastic to Lloyd and me. And many other children are having treatment here.

They weighed Lloyd, took his temperature and blood pressure, and then explained they'd insert a needle into his hand to take blood.

They know this as IV- intravenous, and it has to stay in his hand for four hours.

When the doctor tried to put the needle into Lloyd's hand, they couldn't find the vein, so they tried several times, and it was getting painful for Lloyd.

They got the needle in, and I felt sad for him; I wish I could have had them for him.

I said, "I wish I could have your needles for you, my darling."

Lloyd replied, "You can, mum, because I could watch you have a tattoo?"

I said, "I can't have a tattoo, Lloyd."

Lloyd replied, "Oh, go on, mum, I'd love to watch you have one done."

I said, "Alright, my darling, just for you, maybe on the weekend."

How could I say no after all he was going through?

After four hours, Lloyd's oncology doctor, Dr English, came to see us to explain many things and told Lloyd he would stay on his blood pressure tablets (Nifedipine) and his steroids, but these have changed to Dexamethasone.

I told Dr English that Lloyd was very sleepy and weak and needed his wheelchair to get around.

So I explained he's eating a lot and getting big; Dr English said that he will while he is on steroids.

I explained this to Lloyd and told him most children get bigger when taking steroids, and Lloyd said he doesn't mind as long as he gets better.

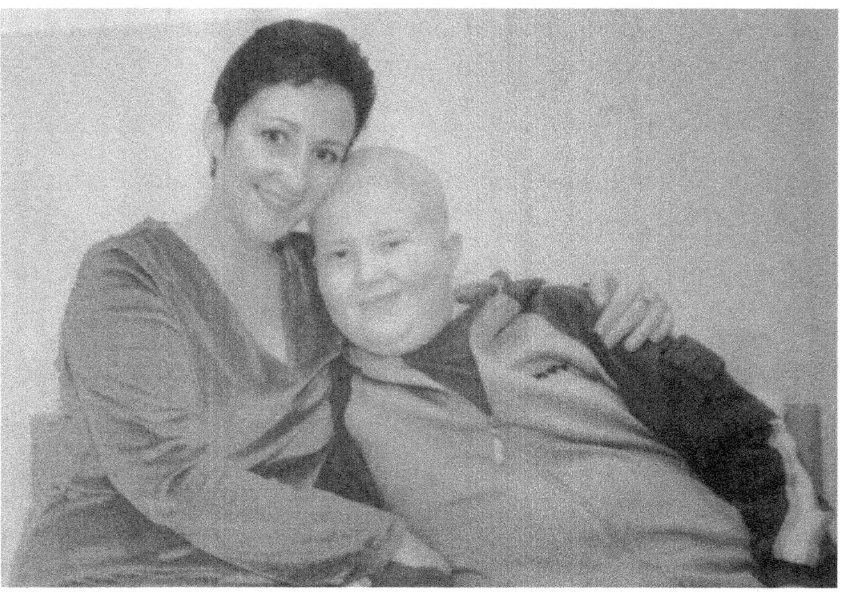

When I hear him say things like that, it breaks my heart.

But he gives so much love to my heart and soul because he's my darling angel, and we love each other.

The weekend arrived, and I promised Lloyd I would have a tattoo done for him, so I made the arrangements.

I spoke to the body artist, explaining several things about Lloyd, and told him what it meant for me to have the tattoo done.

The body artist allowed us to have a private sitting in the tattoo parlour.

Here I am, sitting in the chair, ready and waiting, but unsure if I can be as brave as Lloyd, but I will try my hardest.

Lloyd and I have decided the tattoo will be of a tiny boy angel, with Lloyd's name at the bottom, because I always call him my darling little angel.

The body artist began with the outlining, and WOW, did it sting?

The tattoo will be under my collarbone near the chest area. Lloyd is holding my hand, just as I always do with his hand.

He could see the pain showing on my face, and he cried and said, "I'm sorry, Mum, I wish I had never asked you to have this done."

I replied, "This is special for me to do this for you, and I wish I could go through everything for you."

Lloyd was alright after, and it had been an experience for him.

Today is Tuesday, 5 September, and Lloyd has had nothing to eat or drink because he's having his operation this morning.

It upsets me, but I can't show it.

Lloyd is fine, and when I ask him if he's okay, he never moans or worries and always says, "I'm fine, mum."

They needed me to sign a consent form again for the operation, and now we are off to the anaesthetist for Lloyd to have the anaesthetic.

And this is dreadful, so I hold his hand and kiss him, and we both say we love each other, and then he is fast asleep.

They have taken Lloyd to the operating theatre, so I sit and wait, for what seems like hours, for the nurse to come and take me to the recovery room.

All I could do was wait and wait and pray to God for my baby to get through this.

At last, the nurse came and took me to the recovery room, and when I got there, Lloyd's eyes were open, and when I went to see him, he was in agony.

He began screaming with the pain, so they gave him more pain relief, and then he settled down after a while.

The doctor came to our room and explained to us that there was a needle in Lloyd's chest, and it needed to stay there for seven days before being removed.

They also gave him a lumbar puncture during the operation, and he has a cut on his neck and chest; they have stitched the wounds with dissolving stitches, which is excellent.

Lloyd has been sleeping for quite a while in the morning and is starting his chemotherapy treatment, so I pray he will feel better tomorrow.

He has been awake most of the night with pain in his back because of the lumbar puncture.

The morning has arrived, and Lloyd is beginning his chemotherapy treatment. He has a plastic tube coming from his chest, and it's connected to a machine controlling the flow of the medicine (carboplatin), lasting for one and a quarter hours.

When this ends, they administer another chemotherapy, a drug they know as vincristine treatment; this only takes a brief time.

After this, they add a substance to flush the system, which gets pushed through Lloyd's bloodstream.

They are giving Lloyd anti-sickness tablets.

They give him tablets, they know as ondansetron, every four hours to stop him from being sick, but he still has a lot of pain in his back after his lumbar puncture.

We are returning home tomorrow.

A nurse will call our house daily to check Lloyd's blood pressure, and I can give him codeine for the pain in his back.

He wants to lie on the settee because he doesn't enjoy moving around much, so I need to monitor his temperature.

If it rises to 37.5, I have to ring the hospital, and if it is 38, we will return to the hospital because it will have to do with the chemotherapy treatment.

It is Tuesday, 12 September, and Lloyd's nurse has come to our house to remove the needle from Lloyd's port.

The needle has been in his chest for seven days now, so I am glad that they removed it because he could feel it when he was turning over in bed, and it was uncomfortable for him.

The nurse has removed the plaster from his neck and needs a blood sample to test for a blood count and to ensure Lloyd's not neutropenic (low blood count), and also checked for haemoglobin and platelets (white blood count).

They need to check this with someone on chemotherapy treatment.

Today is 13 September, and Lloyd has to go to the Royal Gwent Hospital in Newport at one o'clock for an MRI scan.

It looks like he will have several more of these MRI scans; I know we need them, but it is a very long time for Lloyd to be lying still all the time.

Nothing is fair, and I'm the one who keeps moaning about things, and Lloyd gets on with it; He has so much courage.

After the first half-hour session in the scanner, they pull Lloyd out for an injection to run dye through his bloodstream.

Again, they had problems finding his veins, and it was hurting Lloyd a lot, so I was getting angry with them for putting him through all this pain.

If they had mentioned the dye injection sooner, I could have put Ametop (deadening cream) on his hands and arms to prevent the pain from the needles.

At last, they could find a vein and administered the dye to Lloyd, which he said was freezing and a little sore as it went through his body.

He was in the MRI scanner for a long time, and because he is always brave, I bought him a gift and took him to McDonald's; he deserves it.

Thursday, 14 September.

And off we go to Llandough Hospital in Penarth near Cardiff to see Lloyd's specialist, Dr English.

I am glad we are seeing him because I'm worried about Lloyd's shunt, as the back of his head is very red, and he's suffering from headaches.

After checking Lloyd's shunt, Dr English told me there was an infection in that part of the head, so he prescribed antibiotics.

Lloyd isn't having carboplatin chemotherapy today, only vincristine treatment, so they inserted another needle in his hand.

You think to yourself, why?

Why do they have to go through all this pain and suffering?

Today, in the oncology unit, I have noticed so many children with different illnesses, all requiring chemotherapy treatment, and every one of them is a happy, brave, courageous child.

So, when I hear somebody moaning about feeling depressed or having a cold, I think to myself, look what these little children are going through, and believe me, they would never moan again.

I have been changing the dressing on Lloyd's port, where they removed the needle, as it has been weeping, so Lloyd has called me Nurse Pike, and he needs to take his antibiotics for seven days.

I don't know what is causing it, but Lloyd has very sore feet, so the doctor has prescribed Daktarin cream to rub on them every day for ten days.

We will see Dr English next Thursday because Chemotherapy treatment is every Thursday for one year, and Lloyd has a blood count to check that the count is okay for Thursday's chemotherapy session.

Thursday, 21 September 2000 and back to Llandough Hospital for more chemotherapy treatment.

They are only giving Lloyd Vincristine again this week, which makes him sick, but he has the ondansetron anti-sickness tablets to combat this.

He also gets sleepy and sleeps for two to three hours throughout the day.

Later, he had a sore throat, and his temperature was 37.3, so he went to sleep. I'll stay by his side to check on him.

I can't leave his side for five minutes, and I don't want to leave his side at all because he is my world, and I am devastated he is going through this.

Lloyd's sore throat is much better today. Thank God. And his temperature has dropped back to normal; I don't want him to have another injection.

The trouble with the chemotherapy treatment is that Lloyd's immune system is low, and he can pick up an infection at any time.

Today is Wednesday, 27 September 2000, and the nurse is coming to our house to take blood from Lloyd's port to see if he will be okay for the chemotherapy session on Thursday.

They need to take blood just before because if the blood count is low, he won't be able to take the chemotherapy treatment.

I have put Ametop cream on Lloyd's chest on his port to deaden the area so the needle doesn't hurt as much going in.

Lloyd's nurse, Gill, pushed the needle into the port and tried to draw blood, but no blood was coming, so she removed the needle and put it back in; this upset

Lloyd.

These ports should work the first time.

Still no blood, and now, Lloyd is getting more and more upset, so I said to Gill, "Just one more time, and if you don't get any blood this time, I don't want you trying again."

So I promised Lloyd this was the last one, and I won't let Gill try again.

When Gill put the needle in for the third time, I didn't know what happened, but Lloyd was screaming in pain, and I felt so hurt because I should have made her second attempt the last one.

I blamed myself for letting her do it for the third time; it devastated Gill. She didn't want to hurt Lloyd because she liked him very much, and Lloyd liked her too.

I hugged Lloyd and told him how sorry I was, and he said, "Don't be sad, mum, it wasn't your fault."

He is such a caring little boy, and I love him.

Lloyd will have his blood taken early Thursday morning at Llandough Hospital to see if he can have chemotherapy treatment.

Lloyd's blood tests have returned, and it's good news that he will have both chemotherapies today, Vincristine and Carboplatin.

When he has both chemotherapies, we are at Llandough Hospital for hours, and it's a long, depressing day for the two of us.

After his chemotherapy treatment, Lloyd felt sick and is taking his anti-sickness tablets; they stop him from being sick, but he still feels sick.

Chemotherapy also gives him a bad tummy, and he feels weak when he walks, but he is emotional today, crying and saying, "I don't enjoy having a tumour, Mum, and I don't think I will get better."

I felt I would burst into tears, but I must not, because I must keep strong.

I needed to tell him the truth about the questions he asked me, so I said, "You are having chemotherapy treatment to shrink the tumour, and then after the chemotherapy treatment, you will need an MRI scan to see what it has done to the tumour because they hope the chemotherapy will shrink it so you will be ready for radiotherapy next year, okay, Lloyd?"

The treatment they gave Lloyd is not a cure, but it's for him to have a longer life expectancy, and yes, I know it's awful that a child has to go through this to prolong his life, but by doing this, there is always hope for a miracle cure.

If Lloyd didn't have chemotherapy treatment, he would only have three months to live without it; I am praying for a miracle cure.

Yet another week has passed, and Lloyd is due for his blood test.

Gill came to our house, and she inserted the needle on her first try, and it pleased me.

Lloyd's blood count was low, and he wasn't well, so a nurse came to our house on Thursday to give him the vincristine drug only because his blood count wasn't good enough for carboplatin.

Lloyd gets tired and doesn't enjoy doing much, so he lies and rests on the settee, and I sit by his side.

When Gill came to take blood this week, she tried three times again, and she thinks the port has moved, so she is taking blood from Lloyd's finger with a finger prick; Lloyd didn't like the finger prick at all.

If only our mums could have our children's illnesses, because it kills me to see him having to go through all this.

Lloyds blood count is low H.B.10.2 (haemoglobin), platelets 65, W. BC.2.4 (white blood cells), neutrophils 0.3.

He can only have Vincristine chemotherapy today, and they are also taking an X-ray to check the position of his port-a-cath.

Luckily, it hasn't moved, so they will administer the vincristine through his port as the treatment always goes into the port on his chest.

If they have a problem getting the needle into the port, they will put it in the vein on his wrist. And this is painful.

Thank God it went into the port. I prayed it would, and I always pray for God to send my Lloyd a miracle.

So they administered the vincristine. Later in the week, I noticed Lloyd was bruising. I think it was low platelets, so I phoned and explained.

Chapter Six.

What's Ahead Of Us?

Thursday, 19 October 2000, back to Llandough Hospital and the usual Thursday routine.

They gave Lloyd Carboplatin and Vincristine today, but he has a lot of pain in his head where the shunt is situated. The doctor examined it and said that Lloyd had another infection, so he prescribed more antibiotics.

After his chemotherapy treatment today, Lloyd was very sick, although he had anti-sickness medication administered through his port with an intravenous.

They did a few blood tests and found they needed to admit him to the hospital for a blood transfusion.

His blood pressure is very high, and he has a temperature of 38 degrees, so we monitored Lloyd all night.

When you visit the hospital as often as we mothers with sick children for chemotherapy treatment, it teaches you a great deal.

They allowed us to be involved in simple tests such as blood pressure, temperature, pulse, and administering medication. You must be involved and be around your child constantly.

Lloyd had a good night's sleep, and the doctor came to check on him. His blood pressure is still high, so the doctor is stopping his steroids and putting him on a higher dose of blood pressure tablets.

I am worried about the doctor taking Lloyd off his steroids, as I believe we should wean him off them, but the doctor took him off them that morning.

The doctor will allow Lloyd to go home today as long as he rests, and I take him to the Royal Gwent Hospital at least three times daily for blood pressure checks.

Yesterday, his blood pressure was 150/110. It's very high, but today it dropped to 145/100.

Later that evening, I took Lloyd to the hospital for a blood pressure check. We sat in the waiting room with a few other children with broken arms and cut knees, but what bothered me was that Lloyd's limbs were in much pain because of the vincristine chemotherapy.

We waited for hours, and we only wanted a blood pressure check, so I went to the reception desk and explained that Lloyd was having chemotherapy and was not feeling well.

Not long after this, they came and put us into a room and took Lloyd's blood pressure.

I said, "Lloyd, I am not putting you through this three times a day."

So, when we returned home, I contacted Llandough Hospital and explained how long we had been waiting. They said they would arrange for the community nurses to visit our house twice daily.

It pleases me now because he can rest. He likes to lie on the settee because he lacks strength and is taking codeine to ease the pain.

Lloyd's eyes look awful; I am worried about him.

I don't like what he's going through, and it's eating me up inside, yet he never complains and says, "I need to lie down, mum." Lloyd never moans.

He slept well and had his blood pressure taken this morning, and his BP was 140/92. And later in the day, his BP was 145/80.

Lloyd seems worse today than he was yesterday; he is weak, and I'm not happy that they have taken him off his steroids.

He has slept most of the day and hasn't eaten anything since coming to the hospital, and he isn't drinking much.

Lloyd is still taking codeine for the pain in his limbs, but had a restful sleep. The nurse came three times today, and I told her how anxious I was about Lloyd and that I'd talk with the doctor.

His nine o'clock BP was 161/83, his afternoon BP was 147/96, and in the evening, his BP was 148/118.

Lloyd is taking 20mg of Nifedipine blood pressure tablets.

He is having chemotherapy treatment today, Thursdays do come around quickly.

They tried to access his port today but couldn't get any blood, and even though the needle entered the correct place, no blood was flowing, so he was having another X-ray.

The X-ray showed that there doesn't seem to be a problem with the port, but they are giving Lloyd his chemotherapy treatment in his hand, which is painful.

I am annoyed with this port because it's proving problematic and never works the first time as it should.

Friday, 27 October, 2000.

Lloyd's BP this morning was 140/100, later, it was 145/105, and the temperature was 37 degrees.

I have taken Lloyd back to Llandough Hospital because I am far from pleased because things are not correct, and I want them to check him over again.

I don't feel I am an overprotective mother, but I know my baby is suffering. He doesn't moan, and I fear he holds his pain not to worry me, so I need to get something done to help him through this.

Dr English, Lloyd's specialist, was not on call, so another specialist, Dr Jenny, came to see him.

Dr Jenny knew quite a bit about Lloyd's illness, so she asked me many questions about how I felt, so I told her I wasn't happy they had taken him off his steroids so quickly instead of weaning him off them.

She agreed and put him back on a higher dose of steroids because he needed a boost.

He wasn't well, so he had 50mg of Hydrocortisone in the evening and 50mg in the morning.

Then, he will have 20mg three times daily until further notice.

They kept Lloyd in hospital overnight because he had chronic pain in his tummy caused by the chemotherapy treatment, so they gave him Lactulose and Genna for his constipation. The constipation caused him much pain.

He has had Paracetamol for his tummy pain, but it had no effect, so they gave him Ibuprofen to ease the pain.

Later today, we are going to the Heath Hospital in Cardiff for an important eye test, and then we will be allowed to go home after this.

Tonight. Lloyd has been sick, and I believe it is because of the Lactulose medicine, as it's sweet and thick, and he still isn't eating or drinking much, and he has a lot of back and tummy pain, so I gave him Paracetamol because I found codeine can cause him an upset tummy with pain.

Lloyds BP today is 120/90, and in the afternoon, 100/70.

Lloyd had some Weetabix cereal this morning, and when he went to the toilet, he had solid stools and felt much better.

It is 31 October 2000, and it's Lloyd's 9th birthday.

He opened his presents with a struggle; it took him ages because he was unwell, but you could see on his tiny face that he was trying to appreciate his birthday.

Later, we had a big white stretch limousine to take him to his birthday party at the Mega Bowl, but he stayed in his wheelchair the whole day.

When we went to the Wimpy bar for his birthday party, he got out of his wheelchair and lay down on my lap, but struggled to blow out the candles on his cake because he felt unwell. He did it later with a struggle.

He couldn't eat any of his party food and had no strength to go around the houses with me for the Halloween trick-or-treat after his party.

And I know this may seem selfish, but I feel so broken-hearted for him. All the other children are running around as usual, but my poor baby boy is suffering.

Lloyd will have an ultrasound scan tomorrow to see why his blood pressure is so high.

His port hasn't worked again today, so they are arranging for Lloyd to have an anaesthetic on Thursday, 23 November 2000, to correct his port. If they can't adjust his port, they will remove it and replace it with a Hickman line on the other side of his chest.

The doctor is putting Lloyd on a different steroid, Dexamethasone, and this will replace Hydrocortisone and will be taken one three times a day for two days, and then one twice daily for five days.

His BP today is 132/98, and later it is 138/100.

Lloyd is now taking Picosulfate for his constipation and is in a lot of pain with his tummy. Lloyd's nurse is coming again today to remove blood to test for his chemotherapy treatment.

It's the same thing every week, taking blood one day, then chemotherapy treatment on a Thursday, and blood pressure checks daily.

I feel so sad for him because it's as if our world has ended, but I must not let it get to me. Lloyd has a lot of courage, and I need to be a stronger person for him.

Lloyd feels better, so I will take him to visit as many places as possible. He already has many lovely gifts, but I can't get him enough and want to keep buying him pleasant things to compensate for his pain.

And when I knew Lloyd would lose his hair due to the chemotherapy treatment, I shaved it short, so when his hair fell out, he wouldn't notice it much.

He's not bothered about losing his hair because he knows it would grow back. One day, somebody shouted to him, "Hey, meatball head." Lloyd just laughed.

Lloyd has a fantastic sense of humour, and we always joke about and have lots of fun when he's feeling okay, but he sleeps a lot.

He is putting on more weight while taking the steroids, but they make him feel better when he takes them, and he sweats a lot when sleeping because of his weight.

Tomorrow we have to go to Llandough Hospital early in the morning. Lloyd needs another operation, but always understands everything they tell him and never moans about having these operations.

Tomorrow is Thursday, 23 November 2000.

They settled us in a room with two beds. Lloyd is in one, and the other is unoccupied, so I have a camp bed by his side in case someone needs the spare during the night.

The anaesthetist came to see Lloyd and explained things. Lloyd said, "I'm getting used to having these operations."

We will go to the theatre this afternoon. The afternoon has arrived, and we are on our way down to the anaesthetist's room.

I hold Lloyd's hand, kiss him and say sweet dreams, my darling, and in no time, he is fast asleep. It always makes me cry when I have to leave him to go for his operation.

While he is having his operation, I would like to buy him a present for when he comes around.

I found a fabulous present for Lloyd. It's a singing clown, the clown has orange hair, and I sat him on Lloyd's bed, ready for when he returned from the theatre.

As time passed, I waited for a call to go to the recovery room, and while waiting, a nurse shouted to me, "Lloyd's back, mum."

I got out of the chair and walked to the corridor, and Lloyd was there, full of smiles.

He said, "Hi mum, we surprised you."

Because Lloyd was so well, and the time it would take to phone me to go to the recovery room, it was quicker to bring him straight to me.

It was a fabulous surprise for me.

Then Lloyd noticed his recent present, the colourful clown, which he loved and cuddled. Lloyd loves cuddly things.

He loves teddy bears, and we are collecting teddies. At the last count, we have 150, all unique shapes and sizes, and we want to get more.

The nurse gave us some excellent news. They had put Lloyd's port back in place, so he didn't need a Hickman line on the other side of his chest.

The port-a-cath had turned, causing the tube to twist. Therefore, it stopped the blood flow, so a new port-a-cath was required.

But Lloyd's stitches on his head and chest were re-cut, so it will take time for them to heal, and the needle will have to stay in place for seven days.

He will have his Vincristine and Carboplatin chemotherapy, the same as every Thursday, and he will go home tomorrow.

I said to Lloyd, "How are you feeling, my darling?"

He answered with his favourite word, "Fine, thank you, mum."

We are off home today, but Lloyd has an awful pain in his leg and says his bones are aching, so I explained to him, as best I could, that it was the Vincristine chemotherapy attacking his limbs.

Lloyd is having difficulty walking, so he's using his wheelchair a lot, but it's hard to get it around our room.

Chapter Seven.

Trying to Keep Things Normal, Hurts.

Lloyd would love to go to school with his friends, but is in a lot of pain, sleeps often, and has his blood taken once a week, plus chemotherapy treatment on a Thursday.

So, I arranged with our local council for a teacher to visit our house for one hour a week.

We knew her as Mrs Park, and Lloyd thought she was great.

Lloyd had a work desk, which he kept neat, with an office chair for himself and a chair for Mrs Park to sit next to him.

When she gave him work to do, he would do it neatly. Mrs Park said Lloyd was a pleasure to teach and liked him very much.

Lloyd would look forward to Wednesday. It pleased me when he showed me the work he had done. I was proud of him.

Then, one day, Lloyd said, "I don't want to do this school work, Mum, because I'm worried I will not know as much as the others in my class when I return to school." And this was bothering him.

I want Lloyd to be happy, have fun and not worry about schoolwork. In my mind, I don't know what the outcome of his treatment will be, but I don't want to say that to Lloyd.

So, the only thing I can do as a mum is to keep things as normal as possible. I explained everything about Lloyd to Mrs Park, and she will keep him updated with what the other children are doing in school.

Lloyd feels better about that, so we are working together. We love having many things to do together and are inseparable.

Thursday 30 November.

The nurse is coming today. She is removing the needle from the port in Lloyd's chest, but first, she will take blood for testing before Lloyd has his chemotherapy treatment.

He's feeling a little better today, still weak with walking difficulties, but feeling better himself.

However, chemotherapy causes several more problems. Lloyd's hands are stiffening, and his fingers lock, so it's difficult to hold a cup, and he can't feel things when he picks them up.

So, I looked into this, and it's because of the vincristine medication. Lloyd now has hand restraints and special fittings for his shoes because the arches of his feet have collapsed.

I have taken Lloyd to a Hydrotherapy pool; this will relax his body. The water is warm, and the physiotherapist will help him move so he doesn't feel pain.

Well, Lloyd loves it.

If he isn't Neutropenic, we can go once a week. Because when you are Neutropenic, your blood count is low, and you are more likely to catch infections. Pools are the worst places for catching infections, germs and bugs.

They are reducing Lloyd's blood pressure tablets from 60 to 40mg and weaning him off his steroids today.

His blood count isn't good. HG 10.3, WC 4.5, Platelets 78, N.1.3, and his blood pressure is 118/78, so they are not giving him any chemotherapy because his platelets are low.

We are on our way home, and Lloyd wants to pop into the Star Inn to see all his friends who raised money for him to have enjoyable times and lovely gifts.

He likes to pop into The Star pub after his afternoon sleep and loves Coke. And I mean bucket loads of Coke. He also enjoys playing pool and the fruit machines. I will let him do anything that he wants.

He is a sensible little boy, and I feel it's giving him a chance of maturity. He enjoys being around adults, and they love having him around because he touches the hearts of everyone, and they are all good to him.

We have such a wonderful family and friends.

I bought a fruit machine for Lloyd and placed it in our living room for him to play on. It's lots of fun and Lloyd's giant money box. It doesn't pay money out, but he still has plenty of fun playing on it.

Christmas will be here soon, and I want it to be great for Lloyd because I have always made his birthdays, Easter and Christmases special.

And since he was a baby, I have always been extravagant with presents. I have captured every occasion by taking hundreds of photographs and filming videos on a camcorder. I need to catch every moment.

Bonfire night, Lloyd wasn't well and didn't feel like going anywhere, so we had sparklers in our front garden. We didn't enjoy it but had fun with the sparklers.

We always looked forward to Christmas and loved to stay at home. There's no place like home.

Lloyd has had his blood count. And on Thursday, he will only have one chemotherapy, Carboplatin and no Vincristine.

His chemotherapy went okay today, but it tires him. He has finished weaning off his steroids. Lloyd has had some pleasant news. He doesn't need chemotherapy until 18 October 2001. And that's good for Lloyd. He needs a break.

We can look forward to Christmas and pray that Lloyd will feel fine. We love the build-up to Christmas.

I enjoy getting his presents and wrapping them. Lloyd also makes Christmas beautiful for me, and his being here is a precious gift.

I have got him some brilliant gifts, and every year, I always make a giant cracker for the dinner table.

Putting the decorations up is also a marvellous time for both of us. And our living room is like Santa's Grotto, with decorations all over the ceiling and walls. And on the fireplace, we have a band of four Santas playing musical instruments. They are Lloyd's favourites.

The Christmas tree we have is my parents, I have always kept it. I also have baubles and the other tree decorations from my parents. And we use these to decorate the tree.

Lloyd made some decorations in school, and we put them on the tree. I will treasure them forever, along with the tiny fairy he made for the top.

We came home from Llandough Hospital after a blood count. And when we arrived home, outside our front door was the most considerable Christmas tree we had ever seen.

Someone had given it to Lloyd as a gift. We couldn't get it through our front door. We later found out it was a gift from the garden centre where my brother works. We had to cut some off the top and bottom of the tree to get it in the house.

At last, after some cutting, pushing, and shoving, we managed to get it into the front living room. Lloyd thought it was fantastic. It was a fabulous gift.

It was the first time we had ever had an actual Christmas tree, and it smelled gorgeous. It filled the entire side of our room, so we used many decorations, and also hundreds of fairy lights.

We needed a step ladder to put the angel on the top. Also, we couldn't use our usual angel because it was too small. So we had to buy a bigger one.

We have always put up our decorations early; we can't wait, and we love Christmas time.

It's 24 December, and Lloyd can't wait to put out a glass of milk and a mince pie for Santa. And also a carrot for Rudolph. Then, once he has done this, he likes to have an early night.

He has put three stockings on the bedroom door handle and two on the fireplace. I stayed in the bedroom with Lloyd until he fell asleep, and then I got busy.

I always go to bed with Lloyd. And this is because I can't bear being away from him. We sleep in together. Then, at 3.30 am, it's Happy Christmas, Lloyd. The earlier, the better.

Lloyd went to his bedroom door and picked up the three stockings bulging with goodies. He cannot stop saying, "Thanks, Santa, thanks, mum." I have it all on video.

And it's great to see him sitting on his bed, opening his stockings. He always appreciates and loves everything he gets.

On our way down the stairs, with a camcorder in hand. We enter our living room, and

Lloyd's face on the video, when he saw the room full of presents and balloons, was something I'll never forget. I love to see him happy. Thank goodness for camcorders, because they will be something I can watch for the rest of my life.

When he walked into the living room, he shouted WOW! "Thanks, Santa, thanks, mum."

He sat on the settee, and I passed him his presents.

After opening several presents, he would say, "You open yours now, Mum." So I did. He used to love seeing me happy and having gifts. He is a loving child. Then he'd finish opening the rest of his presents.

Lloyd always appreciated everything he had and would open the smallest first, leaving the bigger ones until last. He always had several big ones.

Later, we would sit at our decorated dinner table, with our posh dinner plates and serviettes. And Lloyd's beautiful centrepiece, which he made for me in Cub Scouts.

It's a Christmas log with a large candle, and it's gorgeous.

Lloyd enjoyed his dinner, although he's not keen on Christmas pudding and custard. He would have a bit of pudding, and I always put money in it like my mum used to do.

He would have a wine glass, which I filled with lemonade, to make it look like wine. He couldn't wait to pull his giant cracker. We would do the small ones first to ensure we had our Christmas hats. And then the giant cracker, which we always kept until last.

In it was a dolphin pyjama case. There were dolphins on the continental quilt cover and pillow set, which he had as a present.

He liked to keep his bedroom nice and tidy with everything in its place. Lloyd is an immaculate person in everything he does.

Lloyd is feeling okay, but still sleeps for two hours a day. He is having an afternoon nap. Later, we hope to visit the Star Inn as they are having a Christmas party for Lloyd and all his little friends.

It's a children's Christmas disco, and for Lloyd, I'm dressing up as Mother Christmas. I have gold tinsel for my hair and a hat.

Later, at the Star Inn, it was great to see Lloyd having fun with his friends, and his best friend, Adam, was there. Well, and to be honest, they are more like brothers.

It was brilliant to see him enjoying himself so much; he has been through such an ordeal. I wish this weren't happening to Lloyd. I have always felt that things happen for a reason, but I cannot understand why he has to suffer such pain.

As Christmas passes, we look forward to New Year's Eve at my brother's house. My beautiful sister-in-law is putting on a delicious spread for us all.

Lloyd is having a sleep before we go. We are not going until 21:00, but only if Lloyd wants to go.

Lloyd has awoken, saying he feels fine and wishes to go to my brother's house for New Year's Eve.

My nephew Robert and his girlfriend, Melissa, are at my brother's for the festivities. Lloyd thinks the world of them. He also has plenty of Coke, so he's happy.

I didn't expect us to be here for long, but midnight is looming, and Lloyd wants to watch everyone celebrating. So I have put a chair on the pavement outside my brother's house so he can watch the fireworks.

My brother lives next door to the Star Inn, and many people exited the pub. And most of them were our friends.

Lloyd loved watching them all singing and dancing when the clock struck midnight. Then the landlady of the Star Inn came out and gave Lloyd a bottle of Tommy aftershave.

A few days before. When we were over at the Star Inn, Lloyd bought a raffle ticket. And the aftershave was a prize in the raffle. It was great for him to have won the aftershave.

It upset me throughout New Year's Eve, with my thoughts about what the future had in store for us. I have to keep strong and as happy as possible for him.

We had a great evening, and then we later went home, leaving all the revellers to their celebrating.

1 January 2001. Lloyd has pain in the back of his head and in his shoulder. I've given him some Paracetamol, and later, he felt better.

The next day, Lloyd had a pain in his chest where they fitted his port-a-cath, plus a sore throat, so I gave him some Paracetamol, but it was still no better. But it was getting late, so I waited to see how he was the following morning.

Lloyd is still unwell, so I'm taking him to Llandough Hospital because his temperature is 37.5. The doctor has examined him and given him a blood test.

When the results came back, they showed that Lloyd's platelets were low, so they gave him an eight-hour blood transfusion and 48 hours of antibiotics because of an infection.

The line in his chest has a bug, and it's going to his neck. It is also in his port-a-cath, so Lloyd is on an antibiotic drip, which he will stay on for 48 hours at the hospital. He's having a regular dose of potassium and magnesium tablets, which are huge. I will break them in half so he can swallow them more easily. They are the size of a ten-pence piece. Lloyd finds it difficult to take tablets.

In addition to the blood transfusion, he needs a bag of platelets. We know the antibiotic they are giving him is Teicoplanin. He has been on this for four days. They gave him another blood test and found the bug was still there.

So, the doctors are changing the antibiotic to Vancomycin, which is given to Lloyd via a drip for seven days.

Lloyd still needs to take the potassium and magnesium in tablet form. It breaks my heart to see Lloyd trying to take them, but he is getting used to them now.

He gets on with it and always does as he's asked without moaning.

Lloyd needs more platelets today, which they give him via a drip, similar to a blood transfusion. The platelets have an orange colour to them.

He is Neutropenic, which means he is prone to infections, so we need to ensure that any visitors he may have are not suffering from a cold or any other viruses.

Lloyd is still taking his blood pressure tablets and is due for his chemotherapy today. But his blood test results show HB 9.6/ platelets 2.1/ neutrophils 0.3.

So, because he is neutropenic, he will not have chemotherapy today. He has to rinse his mouth out daily with mouthwash to keep his mouth germ-free. And it tastes awful?

He also needs to take Nystatin drops in his mouth after every meal to prevent any bacteria. What is my little darling Lloyd going to go through next? It's breaking my heart.

By now, it feels like we have been in the hospital for months, and I sleep by his side on a camp bed. He doesn't mind being in this ward, and he likes it if we are in the adolescents' room if the children's wards are full.

Lloyd enjoys being around older people, and this ward is for those over twelve; he thinks it's cool because he's only nine.

They allowed us home today, but Lloyd still needs to take his tablets. Thank God the bug has cleared. He is due for another blood test, which is now every Wednesday, and this ensures he is ready for chemotherapy on Thursday.

No chemotherapy again this week. Lloyd's blood count is low, HB 9.8/ WC 2.6/ Platelets 1.69/ neutrophils 0.4.

Lloyd woke up through the night with terrible pain in his tummy. He often gets pain there because of constipation caused by the chemotherapy.

Lloyd hasn't had chemotherapy for two weeks. But yesterday's blood count was fine. So, he will have reduced carboplatin today.

It's 9 February 2001, and today we are going to London for a special day out for a special boy. We went on the London Eye (Millennium Wheel), and the view of

London was breathtaking.

We also visited Madame Tussauds and the famous Harrods Store, where Lloyd bought some strawberries and a toy rabbit which moves just like a proper one.

The London underground was an experience. We didn't like it that much. But the London bus was brilliant fun, and we enjoyed our day.

12 February 2001. Lloyd's having an MRI scan today to see what has happened since his chemotherapy.

The nurse is coming to take blood first and is leaving the needle in his chest for them to put dye through for the MRI scan. It's better than Lloyd having to have another one in his hand.

We are going to the University Hospital of Wales for the scan at 11.15 am. Lloyd is getting used to these scans, but they are not a pleasurable experience; Lloyd never moans.

While in the waiting room, we sang a funny song I used to sing as a child, and Lloyd thought it was fabulous fun.

We went in for the scan, and they supplied earplugs because we were in the room for a long time. I always hold Lloyd's leg so he knows I am with him.

Time is going on, and we take each day as it comes. Lloyd needs platelets again, but they couldn't get blood from his port-a-cath, so they sent us for an X-ray. The X-ray was fine, and another nurse got blood from the port-a-cath.

Lloyd had a terrible headache last night and can't hear very well. So I checked with the doctor, and he said it had all to do with the pressure in his head.

22 February 2001. Lloyd is not having chemotherapy today. He has a low blood count. The specialist wants to see us about the results of the MRI scan.

Whenever I have to talk about the results, I get a terrible feeling. Why? I don't know, but I always know what they will tell me.

The play teacher has taken Lloyd to the playroom for a while so the specialist could have a private word with me. I sat and gripped my hands as tight as I could as he explained that the chemotherapy hadn't worked as they had thought.

They thought the chemotherapy would shrink the cancer, so the radiotherapy would have a better chance of getting to the tumour. But it had only stopped the cancer from spreading any further, and everything had remained the same.

My poor darling Lloyd has gone through the pain and discomfort for nothing; I am devastated.

They have now said that we have to go to the Royal Marsden Hospital in London for radiotherapy for six weeks. They need to plan with the radiologist because it is high radiotherapy, and they will let us know as soon as possible.

And so they called Lloyd back into the room to explain that he was going to London and that his chemotherapy had finished. It thrills him about this.

They told us to find accommodation outside the hospital because they would classify us as outpatients once a day for six weeks. So I made Lloyd happy by telling him we would return to the London Eye and Madame Tussauds.

And so I thought, until we return to London, let's have fun. So we visited Bristol Zoo. We had a wonderful time.

One day, we were in a taxi, and alongside us at the traffic lights was a beautiful green vintage-looking car. And on the side was written Celtic Manor Hotel. Lloyd thought it was splendid.

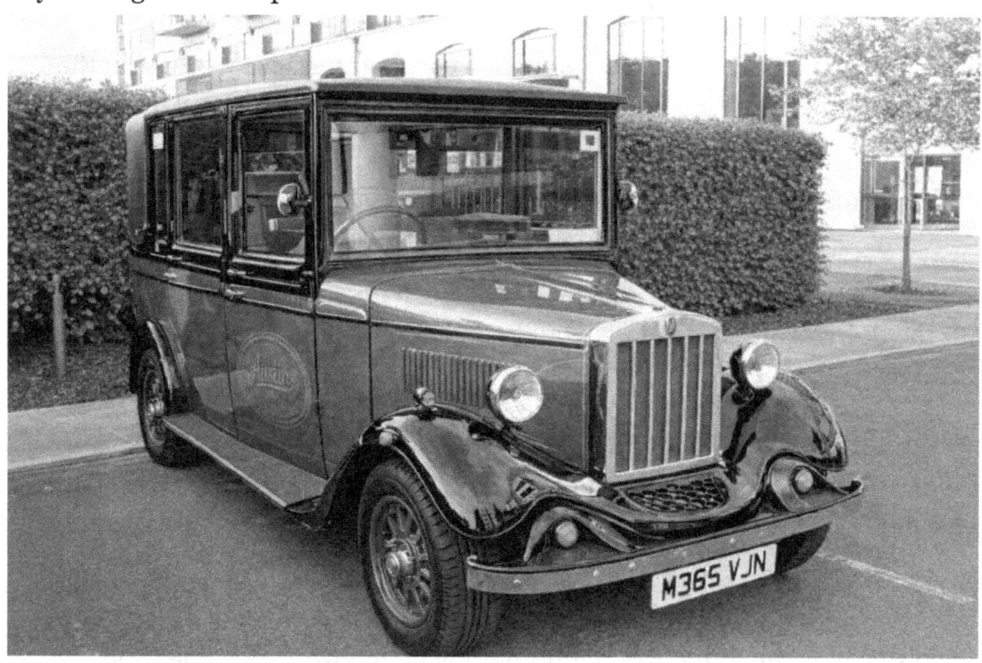

Lloyd's favourite car. The Asquith

So, when we returned home, and Lloyd was having his two-hour sleep, I phoned the Celtic Manor Hotel and spoke to a lovely lady named Catherine.

When I gave her my name, she replied, "Are you Lloyd's mum?" Her mother is one of the nurses who come to our house for his blood pressure check.

The Celtic Manor is a large hotel in Newport, and it isn't far from where we live, so Lloyd doesn't have a long way to travel.

I booked a room for the next night and asked this lovely lady if the vintage-style car could pick us up, and Catherine said they knew the car as the Asquith.

And when Lloyd awakes, I will tell him we will stay in this posh hotel and that we can go swimming. But I will not inform him about the car coming to pick us up.

 I will keep that as a surprise.

The following morning, there was a knock on the door. A smartly dressed chauffeur had arrived in the Asquith car, which Lloyd had seen the day before. You should have seen his face. A wonderful smile beamed right across it.

When we arrived at the hotel, we couldn't believe our eyes. It is fantastic. Lloyd said it was like going abroad, but only down the road.

Lloyd knows what it is like to go abroad. The two of us went to Spain for a week when he was five years old.

We had a splendid time at the Celtic Manor, and everyone was fantastic. We did a lot of swimming. Lloyd loved to swim, and the pool was gorgeous, with stars on the ceiling.

Lloyd also enjoyed the jacuzzi. He loves the water and has gold medals for swimming. I am so proud of him. Very proud in many ways.

He was a proper little gentleman at the hotel and told me to take my elbows off the table. The following morning after our swim, the Asquith car was there to take us home.

I promised Lloyd that one day we'd return to this beautiful hotel.

The phone rang this morning, and we have to go to Llandough Hospital to see Dr Sarong, the radiology specialist, on 15 March 2001.

Dr Sarong explained that the machine they would use for Lloyd's radiotherapy at the Royal Marsden Hospital in London had a problem.

So it would be three weeks before we could go there. Dr Sarong said that Lloyd needed radiotherapy immediately because of how aggressive his tumour's growth was.

He has planned for us to go to the Velindre Hospital in Cardiff instead for treatment. Lloyd will have eight weeks of radiotherapy, two of which will be to prepare a mask.

It disappointed him that we weren't going to London, but he understood the reason.

We will travel to Velindre Hospital for radiotherapy every day for six weeks, starting from 19 March 2001.

Chapter Eight.

Mums Need To Try More.

I have looked into Lloyd's condition and found a great deal about his tumour, and the one piece of information I found hurt like nothing else.

My nephew scoured the internet and found a book which explained Lloyd's tumour.

It stated that anyone diagnosed with a pilocytic astrocytoma typically survives for about two years. There is a machine known as a gamma knife, which directs a laser beam at the tumour to break it up, and it has had some success.

So I wrote to the hospital in London.

I also paid for Lloyd's MRI scans and sent them with a full explanation of the treatment he has already had for his tumour.

I thought the Gamma Knife laser sounded ideal, so I read about it.

So, I waited patiently for a reply, and a week later, I received a letter. The content of which was devastating.

They said they were sorry, but because of how large the tumour is, the surrounding cancer, and the area of the brain it is in, the use of the gamma knife would be futile.

I was not giving up, and I wrote letters and sent them to America, Canada, Australia, and many unfamiliar countries, as well as specialists worldwide, whose answers were the same.

So I spoke to Dr Sarong about Lloyd's radiotherapy and told him I had written to many hospitals about the gamma knife, but they had all written the same reply.

Dr Sarong told me that if we tried radiotherapy, it might shrink the tumour and give Lloyd another five years to live.

I have to agree to the radiotherapy, although I feel Lloyd has been through enough.

Radiotherapy isn't as bad as chemotherapy; the side effects are nowhere near disagreeable, so I had to decide what to do, and I agreed on the radiotherapy.

My Lloyd is such a special boy and a fighter.

19 March 2001. Today is Lloyd's first visit to the Velindre Hospital for a mask fitting for radiotherapy.

We went into a room, and they explained what they would do. They showed Lloyd some plaster, which they dipped in water to place on his face to make a mould.

They let Lloyd feel the plaster, and he put some on his hand and then lay on a bed with no pillow because he would have to lie flat during the treatment.

They put the plaster over his face, and it only took seconds to set

When they removed it, it was in the shape of Lloyd's face; he thought it was funny, so they gave him some plaster to take home, and when we got home, I thought it would be fun for Lloyd to make a mould of my face.

He had lots of fun doing the mould; I wish I could have all his treatment for him.

It's awful that he needs to go through all of this.

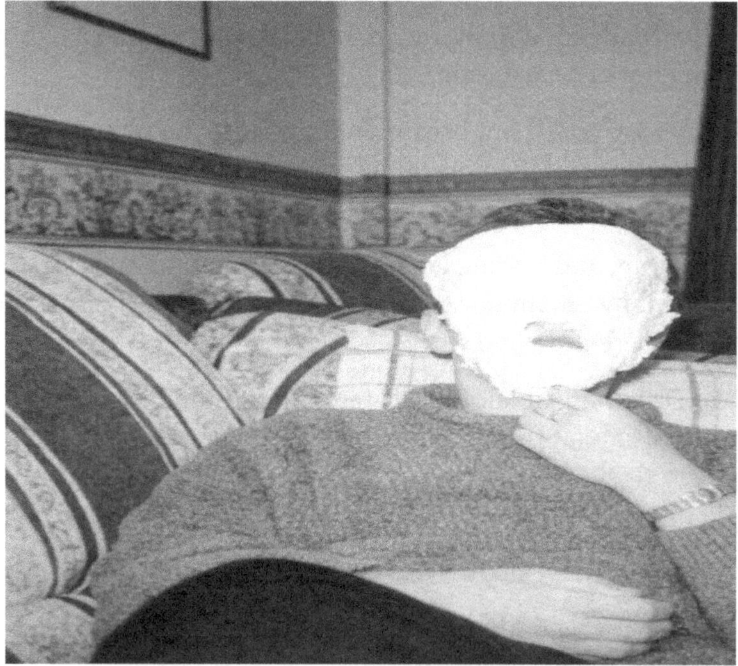

Me, Lloyd's mum, with a plaster mould on my face.

On Wednesday, we are returning to the Velindre Hospital for another sitting, and today, Lloyd has to lie flat on the bed because his mask is ready.

The mask is clear, covers his face and the side of his head, and only has gaps for his mouth and eyes.

We have to go into an unfamiliar room for Lloyd to have X-rays done on his head because they want to direct the radiation to three places: on both sides of the head and the middle.

They call the X-ray machine a simulator, and this is because it resembles the machine Lloyd will be on for the radiotherapy.

The room he will go to for the radiotherapy is down a long corridor, and then you turn left and right. The passage is a zigzag because of the radiation.

They showed us the cameras and televisions, and a nurse lay on a bed so we could see her on a monitor.

They told us that if it frightened Lloyd at any point during the treatment, he could press a button, which he would be holding.

Lloyd said, "I'll be fine, I won't be pressing the button."

They also said Lloyd could play his favourite music during treatment.

So he chose the group we know as "S Club 7."

They will print a poster of S Club 7 and superimpose a picture of Lloyd's face on it.

Every day for six weeks, Lloyd will put a sticker on the poster, and they will also give him sweets; at the end of the six weeks, he will have a present for his courage.

Today's X-ray calculates where to direct the radiation. It will take a long time, and he needs to wear the mask to mark it.

The mask looks frightening, but Lloyd has such bravery and patience, so when they explain, it interests Lloyd about what they will do.

Lloyd knows that when he is having his radiotherapy, I am only at the end of the corridor watching him on the monitor.

We have a lot of trust in each other.

After this session, we don't have to come again until 2 April 2001.

I can't believe what happened today; Lloyd fell over and twisted his ankle, so we have been in the casualty department all afternoon, as if he isn't going through enough.

I wish these things would happen to me and not to Lloyd because he is in a lot of pain and has to wear a crepe bandage and keep his foot up.

I feel so hurt and keep saying to myself, WHY?

He has done nothing to deserve this and is such a loving little boy; Lloyd still sleeps two to three hours daily.

The days pass, and Lloyd's ankle feels a little better, but he has no strength because the chemotherapy is causing weakness in his feet, but we can get him around in his wheelchair.

Today, I am taking Lloyd to the Celtic Manor Hotel to stay the night because he loves it there. They are collecting us in a Bentley car with a chauffeur. I have taken many photographs.

Later today, we are having a mud bath. Lloyd and I have always wanted to do it, and it will be great fun. And this afternoon, we will drive around the golf course in a buggy, which will also be good.

Lloyd's foot is getting painful again, so I think he will have problems with it.

I need to take Lloyd on a few enjoyable days out before he starts his treatment, and so today, we are going to the fair at Tredegar House. Lloyd loves the fair, but he doesn't go on any of the fast rides any more.

And this was his own decision, but we still had fun and won many things in the different stalls.

It's three o'clock in the afternoon of 2 April 2001.

Lloyd needs another X-ray of his head to ensure the markings on his face mask are correct. The nurse will come to take blood from his port-a-cath later, because his magnesium level is low, and they will test it.

She had problems drawing blood from his port-a-cath, and it was painful for Lloyd; the nurse did not understand why.

The nurse has decided not to try another area in the port-a-cath and will leave it until a future day, but Lloyd needs one more X-ray on 9 April 2001, and he will start his radiotherapy treatment on 11 April 2001, which will continue until 25 May 2001.

So, I am taking Lloyd to our caravan in Devon, and I will spoil him as much as possible over the weekend.

It is 11 April 2001, and this is Lloyd's first day of radiotherapy. We went into a room, and Lloyd lay on the bed. He had a gigantic machine around him, and they placed his mask on his face.

The mask has holes on the sides to attach to the bed, stopping Lloyd's head from moving during the treatment. Lloyd, wearing the mask while fastened to the bed, was upsetting for us. But he has to keep still.

Lloyd said. "Don't worry, Mum, I'll be fine. You can go now and watch me on the monitor."

So I kissed him, put on S Club 7 for him to listen to, and left the room. I went to another room to watch him on the monitor.

The radiologist set the machine up on one side of his head, entered the room and pressed the operation buttons.

She then returned to the machine, advanced it by remote control to the other side of the head, re-entered the room and pressed the buttons to operate the radiation.

Then, the last one was at the top of Lloyd's head, so she followed the same procedure, moving the machine. She then returned to the room, pushed the button for the radiation and at last, they finished it.

I was watching all this on the monitor screen. Lloyd never moved a single muscle throughout his treatment.

They are allowing me to see him now. And they are letting Lloyd move the machine away with the remote control. He enjoys doing that, and they have removed his mask. I asked Lloyd how it felt. And guess what he said? "I'm fine, mum." His favourite words.

They have given Lloyd a sweet and a sticker to put on his chart. They will repeat this procedure every Monday to Friday (not weekends) until 25 May 2001 at the Velindre Hospital, Cardiff, Wales. Everyone has been very good to us.

12 April 2001. When Lloyd's radiotherapy has ended today, we have to go to Llandough Hospital for him to have blood taken to check his magnesium level.

They are also flushing his port-a-cath by placing a needle into his chest where the port-a-cath is and then flushing saline through the tube to prevent blockages and infections in the line.

Lloyd is still taking nifedipine blood pressure tablets and must continue to take these until after the radiotherapy.

Today is Good Friday, and Lloyd woke up this morning with a pain in his sprained foot. I believe Lloyd will always have persistent problems with this foot now, but some days are worse than others.

No radiotherapy today because it's Saturday, and it's great to have a break from it.

15 April 2001. Easter Day today. So, Lloyd is having an Easter Egg hunt in our home, starting from the bedroom.

He will have a piece of paper with a clue as to where to find the first egg, and when he discovers it, another clue will help him find the next one.

I have made 19 clues, and there will be presents and eggs.

Somehow, I will push Lloyd around the house in his wheelchair because he is too ill to walk.

So, I place the Easter eggs in the microwave, fridge, oven, and washing machine. Under the stairs, all over the place. Lloyd is having splendid fun. He had a fabulous morning.

The Asda Company are giving Lloyd a special treat. They invited us and told us the time to go there. My nephew Robert, who works at Asda, is dressed up as a rabbit. All the management gathered around Lloyd as he rode an electric scooter supplied by Asda.

They gave Lloyd Easter eggs and cuddly toys, which he collects (he has over 300 cuddly toys), and then Robert went up to Lloyd, dressed as a rabbit.

Lloyd said. "Hiya, Rob, I know it's you. I can tell by your walk?"

Everybody burst out laughing. It was a fabulous day.

A few days on and today is 18 April 2001.

After Lloyd's radiotherapy, he needs another X-ray, but this takes a long time. And I feel so sad for him because after lying still for the radiotherapy, he has to do it again for an X-ray on his head.

They need to ensure that the radiation is accurate when applying it to his head.

They need another X-ray tomorrow after his radiotherapy, so I believe a nice treat is in order, and I've booked a stay at his favourite place, The Celtic Manor Hotel, and I've asked if they will send the Asquith car to collect us.

The Bentley is beautiful, albeit a little boring and not much fun, but the Asquith is old and bumpy, and we have fun riding in the back.

So, I will book two nights and spoil him as much as possible. We will go to The

Velindre Hospital from the hotel.

A week of radiotherapy has passed, so I'm going to surprise Lloyd.

I have booked the Coca-Cola room at the Alton Towers Hotel and Theme Park because Lloyd adores Coca-Cola and drinks gallons of it.

I've had balloons put in the room and a message displayed on the television system saying, I love you, Lloyd, love from Mum.

Lloyd doesn't know what to expect when we go to Alton Towers.

We have arrived at the hotel, and Lloyd thinks it's fabulous because the lift is like something out of a film and plays spooky music.

When we went to our hotel room, Lloyd couldn't believe his eyes because everything was Coca-Cola-themed; it was fabulous. The fridge in the room was full of Coca-Cola and a Smartie sweet machine.

You normally put 20p in the machine, but they made it cost-free. So every time you turned the handle, the Smarties would come out, and there was a card telling you how to find hidden treasure in the room.

Lloyd hunted around the room and found a cardboard treasure chest, and inside were games. It was splendid fun.

We had a fabulous evening in the hotel arcade and spent a lot of money. We bought a teddy, a drinking cup, and many other goodies.

The following morning, I noticed hair on both sides of Lloyd's head had fallen out overnight, and it was all over his pillow. Lloyd's hair had grown back and looked nice again after the chemotherapy. But now it's all coming out again. Lloyd never complained about it. He never complains.

We went to breakfast, and Lloyd saw an enormous teddy bear sitting at our breakfast table. They know the bear as Alton Bear. Lloyd had fun with him and enjoyed himself. Then we went off to the funfair.

We are having a fantastic time and winning many teddies on the fun stalls. We had a fabulous time, but we are returning home this afternoon because Lloyd has radiotherapy tomorrow. Lloyd's nurse is coming today to flush his port-a-cath. She came and thank God, Lloyds port-a-cath worked the first time.

Several more days have passed, and Lloyd's hair has fallen out all around the side and across the front; he has a bit of hair on the top, but he isn't complaining. I am proud of my brave little soldier.

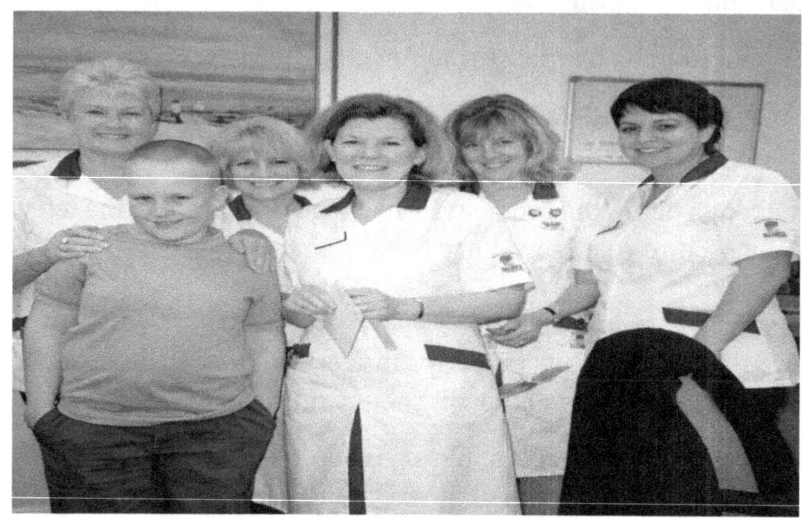

Lloyd with the nurses at Velindre Hospital.

18 May 2001.

After today's radiotherapy treatment, we went to a beauty salon near our home, and Lloyd had his two thumbnails painted. I also had mine painted. Lloyd has Winnie the Pooh on one thumb and Tas, the Tasmanian Devil, on the other nail.

Today, we went to the Millennium Stadium to watch the Welsh rugby team training. Lloyd had his photograph taken with Graham Henry (coach), Neil Jenkins (outside half) and all the other members of the Welsh team.

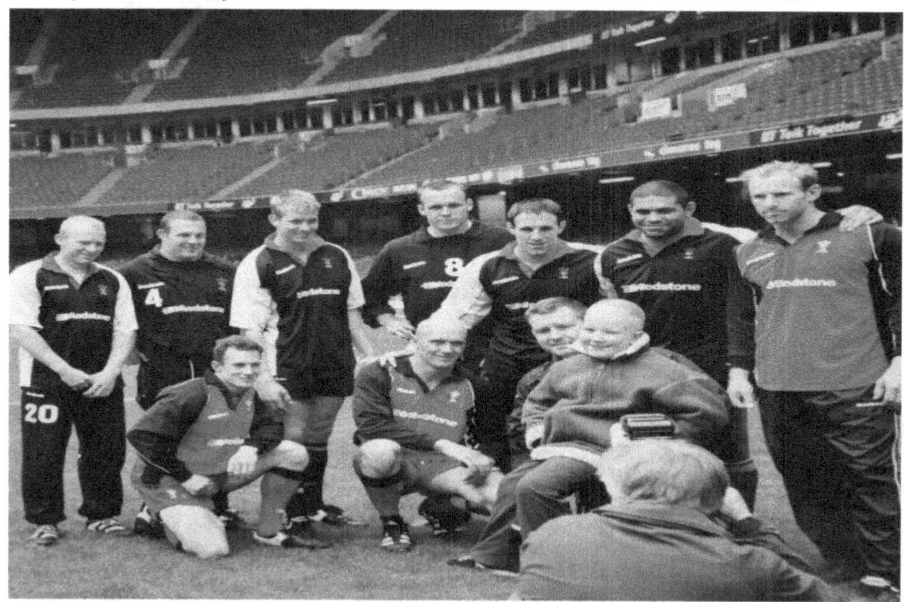

Lloyd with several members of the Welsh rugby team.

Lloyd was chatting with them all and had an enjoyable time. And he had loads of photos taken.

Tomorrow. We are returning to the Millennium Stadium to watch the Wales vs Barbarians match. We are watching the game from a Hospitality Suite, and I have bought Lloyd a funny Welsh hat, a rugby teddy bear and a Welsh flag.

Today is the day. It is Lloyd's first time at a rugby game or any other match. He has never fancied playing rugby or football, but is looking forward to it today. I have my camcorder with me, so I can record everything we do and everywhere we go.

I believe you must have plenty of photographs and videos to cherish the moments.

As the day continued, Lloyd was having a fantastic time, and he enjoyed every minute; he loved it.

Back to radiotherapy today, and not long left to go. But these six weeks of travelling back and forth every day have taken their toll and have been difficult.

So, at the weekend. I am taking Lloyd to the Celtic Manor Hotel again; He deserves it.

We are now at the Celtic Manor and having a fabulous time. In the evening, they surprised us. Three world champion snooker players were there, who gave Lloyd their autographs.

Tomorrow. We are going to the swimming pool, and my sister-in-law, Mandy, is coming to meet us for lunch in the leisure cafe. And then we'll return for radiotherapy the next day.

Not long now, and we are counting down the days. Lloyd will have a present when his six weeks are over.

Just a few more to go now, 5-4-3-2-1.

And that's it, the last day today. Hooray for Lloyd.

When we finished today's radiotherapy, the radiology staff gathered around Lloyd after his session and said it's been fabulous to have known such a lovely, well-mannered little boy.

And they commented on his bravery and gave him his chart, with lots of sweets and a present.

The present was a virtual reality steering wheel with an eyepiece. It makes you feel like you are driving. Lloyd said thank you, and it was fantastic to have known them all.

My gift to Lloyd was to take him to his favourite place, you guessed it, the Celtic Manor Hotel, for the night.

At the Celtic Manor today, Lloyd had a splendid surprise. Terry Matthews, the billionaire owner of the hotel, was having breakfast and invited Lloyd to meet him.

We sat at his table, and he was lovely and chatty. His words were, "Lloyd, be persistent because persistence is what's got me to where I am today. Be persistent, Lloyd."

He then gave Lloyd his autograph, and we had a photograph with him. Lloyd thought he was a fabulous man.

26 May 2001. We are going on a trip to Devon in our caravan. Lloyd loves Devon, and we are going for the weekend. We need to spend as much quality time together as we can.

Lloyd hasn't been to school since July 2000 due to being unwell while having his treatment. We are inseparable, cherish the time we have left, and love each other so much.

I am trying to do so much for him. Lloyd has been in a helicopter and visited a police station. And they took us out in a police-armed response vehicle with the sirens blaring.

They also put on a show for us with a police dog and his handler. We took plenty of photographs and videos of everything. Lloyd has also been in limousines, and I intend to do more with him. We need quality time together.

Back home. And we are off to a place they know as Barry Island in South Wales. We are going on a train. Lloyd loves the train.

We sat on the train, trundling away, when it stopped to pick up some people at a station. Lloyd said, "Wouldn't it be funny, Mum? If the train went back to where we just came from?"

I laughed and said, "It won't do that. The train's picking up people, and then we will go to Barry Island?"

Well, guess what? Yes, it happened. The train picked up the people and returned to the place where we had just come.

I looked at Lloyd and said, "How did you know that would happen?"

He replied. "I don't know. I was only joking, mum."

So we had to get off the train and get another one. We changed trains, and all we could do was laugh.

Once we got to Barry Island, we had a fabulous time. Lloyd loves the arcades, and we won many teddy bears and cuddly toys. I always try hard to give him some toys.

We have had such a splendid day; we are going again tomorrow. But this time, we will make sure we catch the correct train.

One afternoon, several days later, Lloyd was in pain with his testicles and felt sick. The doctor said it was the side effects of the radiotherapy. It can cause sterility, but that is the least of our problems.

I don't want him to feel pain; he goes through enough.

He's weak and can't walk very well.

Lloyd feels better today, so I am taking him to the Celtic Manor golf course and driving range to hit some golf balls around.

We received a letter from the hotel's owner, Terry Matthews, stating that Lloyd should visit the golf club and use the driving range. So we did, and we had marvellous fun.

The next day, I took Lloyd to the Hilton Hotel in Newport, South Wales, for a swim. I prefer to take him to hotel swimming pools because they are quieter than public baths. We had a splendid afternoon and plenty of fun.

Today, we are going to Techniquest in Cardiff. It was interesting, and then we visited a pub they know as the Sports Cafe for lunch, which was very enjoyable.

And at the weekend, we will take Lloyd to our caravan in Devon for a week and have plenty of pleasant trips out and about the countryside.

We are having lunch at the Bideford Arms and then off to the dinosaur park; this is brilliant fun, with a fabulous train ride. It stops in an old gold mine. A blast of water comes splashing over, and you get soaking wet. Lloyd loved it.

The next day, we went to a pub they know as the Pack-O-Cards, then later to an amusement park they know as Once Upon A Time. That was brilliant fun.

Tomorrow we are going to Watermouth Castle. And this was another fun place with rides in a place called Gnomeland. Lloyd had a gnome from the Gnomeland mine. We also had a gnome to hang in our bedroom window at home to bring us luck.

We are off to Ilfracombe today; it has plenty of arcades there for Lloyd to enjoy himself and win lots of teddies, and then we can sit by the harbour with a bag of chips and a tin of Coca-Cola for Lloyd.

It is 30 June 2001. We are going home today; we had a splendid time in our beautiful caravan.

This evening, we'll have another special treat. We will go to Perfect Pizza. They have invited Lloyd to help make some pizzas. He made six pizzas and enjoyed himself doing it. He even had a Perfect Pizza hat to wear when making them. And this was another fun time for him. The following day, my brother and his friend came to our home on their motorbikes to take Lloyd to McDonald's.

He sat on the back of my brother's motorbike, and off they went to McDonald's; I followed behind in the car with my sister-in-law. Lloyd was going on the back of the bike, and I was nervous, but my brother was careful.

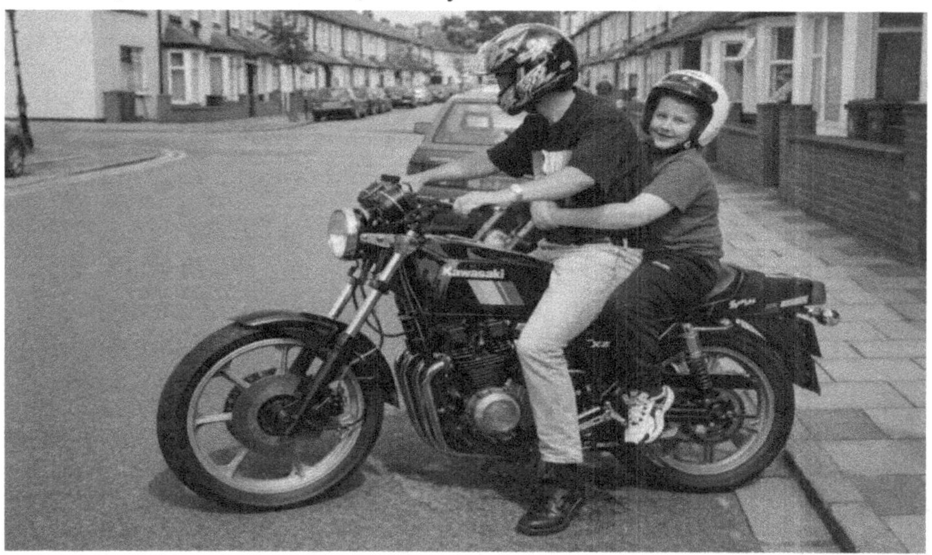

Lloyd on the back of his uncle's motorbike.

I filmed them going to McDonald's. When we arrived, Lloyd had his favourite meal, chicken nuggets with French fries and a Coke, and then we returned home.

Lloyd is a grown-up boy in his own way. He's a little adult, so I call him my little man. His shoe is size 7, and Lloyd is over five feet tall. He's gorgeous, and everyone loves him.

He touches everyone's hearts, even babies. When Lloyd sees a baby, he will go to them, and they love him. They giggle and smile, and he holds their hands.

It's so amazing to see. Lloyd is a beautiful young man and always will be.

We are going to the Donington motor racing track to see the sports cars. Lloyd enjoyed it, but it was loud.

Tomorrow, we are going for a ride in an articulated lorry. It's the largest lorry Lloyd has ever seen. Then, in the evening, we are going to a Skittles night that our friend Dorothy (Dot) organised. It is to raise money for Lloyd.

If not for our brilliant friends and family, and all the people who contributed, we would never have been able to do what we have. We cannot thank them enough for their generosity, and if everyone in the world were like them, what a beautiful world it would be.

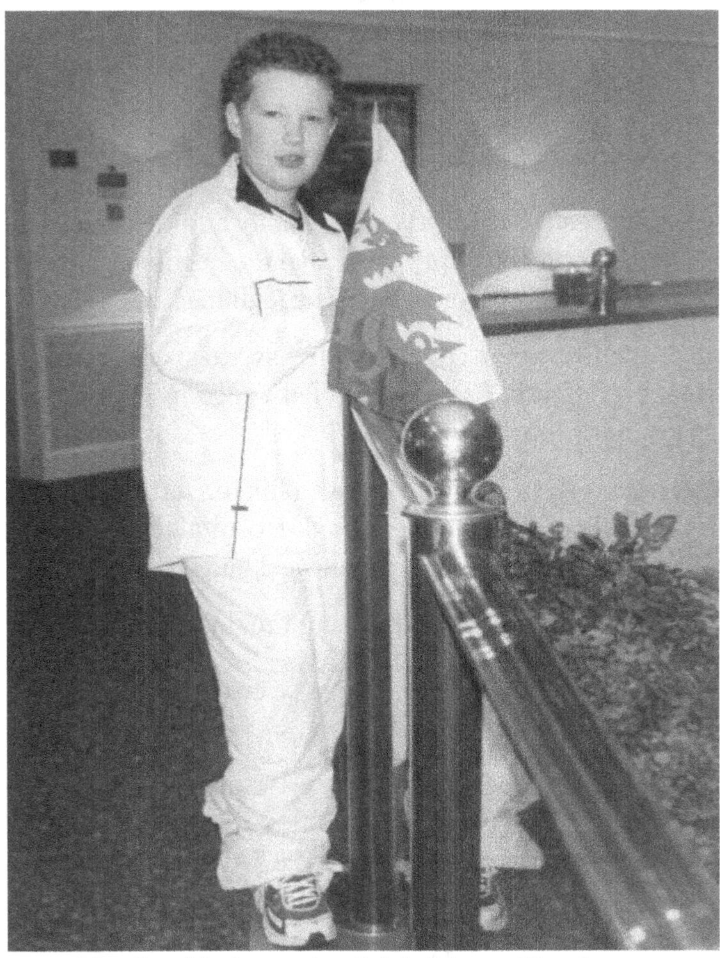

Lloyd at his favourite Celtic Manor Hotel.

Chapter Nine.

What Else Is Ahead Of Us Now?

04/07/2001, 04.50 am. Lloyd woke with a terrible tummy ache this morning and was sick. I contacted our local doctor, who said Lloyd's got a stomach bug.

However, I was not satisfied with the diagnosis, so I took Lloyd to Llandough Hospital to see his oncologist.

The Oncology ward nurses inserted a needle into Lloyd's port-a-cath and removed some blood for testing blood cultures. I don't believe the news. It's terrible, and I think Lloyd has a bug in the port-a-cath line again.

We have given him antibiotics known as Ticoplanin, which he needs to take for one week. Lloyd has been sick and has a temperature of 37.3. He hasn't been passing solids for a week and has constipation.

They've told us we must stay in the hospital overnight, and we can return home tomorrow if Lloyd's temperature decreases.

The doctors have agreed that Lloyd can go home, and the nurse will call at our home from Monday to Friday. They will leave the needle in Lloyd's port-a-cath and administer the antibiotics once daily through his line.

If Ticoplanin doesn't work for Lloyd, he will have to spend a week in the hospital and take a different antibiotic, called Vancomycin, daily. So, I'm praying the Ticoplanin works for Lloyd.

Lloyd is unwell and feeling sick. I have given him an anti-sickness tablet. It is Sunday today, and we must go to Llandough Hospital for Lloyd's antibiotic injection because the nurse doesn't call on weekends.

It worries me because Lloyd isn't eating, but the doctor said he'll be good if he drinks plenty of water, so I will try to persuade him to eat little bits of his favourite food.

Lloyd loves mashed potatoes with spaghetti hoops and mixes them himself.

Lloyd also enjoys toast and Marmite cut into soldiers. It pleased me this morning at breakfast because he had two pieces of toast with Marmite.

Today, he is continuing with his Ticoplanin antibiotic, and the seven-day course will finish on Thursday, which is fantastic.

Lloyd had some pie and chips from the chip shop. He enjoys dipping his chips in the pie. I always eat whatever he leaves over. We must do this because the meal is far too much for one person to eat.

It still worries me that Lloyd hasn't had a bowel movement.

It's 12/07/2001, Lloyd's last day on antibiotics, and they are removing the needle from his port-a-cath. It pleases me as it irritates him at night because Lloyd sleeps on his front.

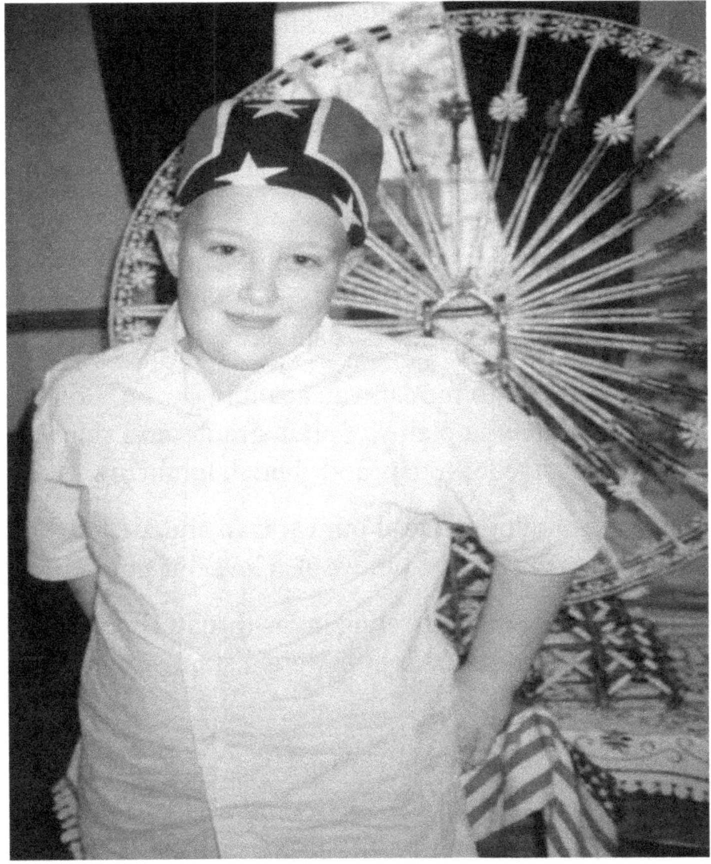

Lloyd wearing his cool bandana.

Several days have passed, and finally, Lloyd has passed solids. I am so happy for him.

Lloyd's nurse is coming today to take some blood to test for cultures to see if the bug has gone from his line.

Thank God the bug is no longer in Lloyd's line. He must have got it in a swimming pool, so we are not swimming for a while. It's better to be safe than sorry.

Lloyd deserves a holiday, so I am taking him to Unity Farm in Somerset to stay in a villa.

We have arrived at Unity Farm, and Lloyd is having a fantastic time at the fair on the rides and in the arcades.

He has found a machine that you put 10p. The wheel turns and throws the 10p into a slot. A different one every time, and then it gives out a ticket. We will save all the machine tickets that it gives out during our holiday. And then take them to the shop and exchange the tickets for something nice.

If we choose something in the shop and don't have enough tickets, we can add cash to make up the difference.

Well, Lloyd is having a fabulous week. And he is wearing a bandana on his head, and it looks great.

Lloyd has used all his tickets in the shop and has a beautiful water feature with fairies. Lloyd appreciates enjoyable things, so I got him another water feature, but this one is a haunted house and plays spooky music.

27/07/2001. And we are off to the caravan again in Devon. Don't forget that quality time is paramount with plenty of photographs and videos. You must make every day special, live for today, and cherish tomorrow.

We have had another fabulous time at our caravan and are heading home sweet home today. We enjoy going away, but we also love our home.

This evening, Lloyd had a strange feeling in his throat. He couldn't explain it. It wasn't sore, but it felt funny, and his eyes were distant with a glazed look about them.

He was making a strange moaning noise as if he were in pain, but it passed after a short while. But I must monitor him.

It happened again today, twice? And this is not right?

Again, it happened while Lloyd was walking. He had to stop because it frightened him. I am taking him to the doctor for a check.

The doctor examined Lloyd and explained that the brain tumour was resting on a nerve behind the optic tract of his eye, and this caused the eye to stare.

The tumour is causing a feeling in his throat. Lloyd is still not eating much food. Oh, please, God, send my baby a miracle. I beg you.

Every night, I pray to God for a miracle for my child.

The Oncology ward at Llandough Hospital has a charitable organisation called

LATCH, which helps families of children ill with cancer, leukaemia, brain tumours and other life-threatening illnesses.

They help in many distinct ways and are taking us on a lovely trip today to Highgrove, the home of Prince Charles, but we are only having a tour of the gardens and the shop he has on his grounds.

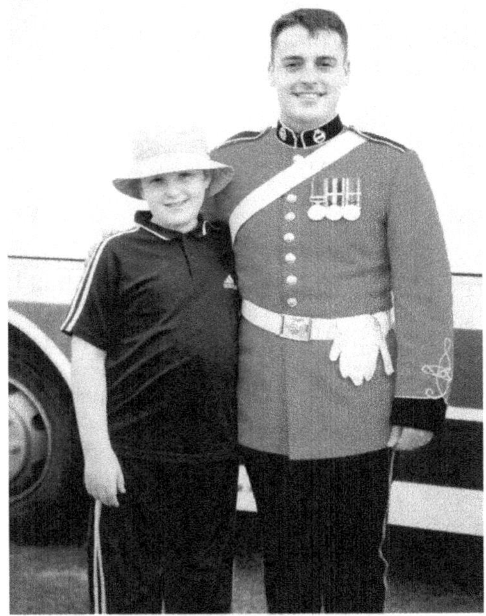

Lloyd with a Guardsman.

We are now on our coach to Highgrove, with several of the Queen's Guards having fun. Prince Charles' garden is organic and beautiful.

The Prince's gardener showed us around the gardens, and then we visited the shop and bought some objects. It upsets me because Lloyd hasn't been feeling well today, but he still fights.

I've noticed Lloyd is finding his vision harder to use, so the chair in our living room must be near the television screen for him to see it.

I have spoken to Lloyd's specialist, who referred us to his colleague at the Royal Gwent Hospital, Newport, near where we live.

We have a date today, and when they test Lloyd, the results concern them.

Terrible news again for us as they are registering my baby as blind. He needs a specialised pair of glasses with orange lenses, which will help Lloyd with the glare of everyday light. He also has a special magnifying glass.

Why, oh why, is this happening to my baby?

Today, I noticed that when Lloyd breaks wind, there is a quantity of clear fluid in his underwear. And this upset him because we can be anywhere when these accidents happen, and he needs to have a change of clothes.

The nurse is coming to flush saline through Lloyd's port-a-cath to keep it clear, so I will hold his hand when they insert the needle, although today, he asked me to do something in the kitchen.

When I returned, he sat on the chair laughing, so I said, "What's the joke then? Are you going to tell me?"

Lloyd replied, "Yes. I've got a surprise for you."

I said, "And what is that then, Lloyd?"

Lloyd replied, "I have had my needle, and the nurse has finished."

I hugged him tightly and said, "What a brave little soldier you are, Lloyd."

The nurse will take a solid sample for testing to check if Lloyd has a problem, but I feel something is wrong.

For a treat today, I am taking Lloyd to Barry Island on the train. He loves Barry Island. We always love a fantastic time and brought home a massive teddy bear.

Lloyd's sample has returned, and it's clear. No bug. So we are off to the caravan again for the weekend to have a splendid time.

He wakes during the night with tummy pain, lasting throughout the day. I am wondering whether the cause of this is stomach wind. Lloyd's stomach seems to have got big. I believe a lack of food may cause this, as he isn't eating enough.

Lloyd's bowel movements are loose but not as bad as diarrhoea. I will try harder to encourage him to eat a little more often.

23/08/2001. A fabulous charity we know as Starlight has offered Lloyd a wish. They allow an ill child to make three wishes, and Starlight will choose one for them.

Lloyd's wish was to visit Disneyland Paris. We had been to Florida before they diagnosed him. But is it difficult to get insurance for a terminally ill child?

The Starlight Charity arranged everything for us, and we are truly grateful. Thank you so much, Starlight, for our brilliant weekend.

When we travelled from Newport to Paddington on the train, Lloyd was sick and had a severe headache. We thought it could have been because he was sitting with his back to the train and travelling backwards.

So, on arriving at Paddington station, we went straight to the first aid station. They let us telephone Lloyd's specialist, who confirmed that travelling backwards was the probable cause of his sickness and headache.

Lloyd felt better after twenty minutes, so we continued to the hotel in London, which Starlight had arranged for us. The hotel was fabulous, and our room was gorgeous.

Inside the room was a welcome letter from the hotel manager, including a box of chocolates. They are kind to us.

Our Eurostar train leaves at 09.30 am. Lloyd thinks the train is brilliant, and so do I. It is a lengthy journey, but we have plenty of sweets, crisps, pop, and other goodies on our trip.

When we arrived at the Paris rail station, our hotel was only ten minutes away, and what a fantastic hotel! They know it as The New York Hotel. It is something else.

Our room is the Presidential Suite.

Mickey Mouse, Pluto, and Minnie Mouse greeted us with all the other Disney characters. It was so touching to see. They were fantastic to Lloyd, and he kept kissing them.

The hotel gave Lloyd a carrier bag. And in it was a Mickey Mouse doll, a photo album, playing cards, a mug and other goodies. They were all so kind to us. Later, we visited Disney Parks and had such a great time.

And this morning, Lloyd is having breakfast with the Disney characters. Starlight arranged this.

The characters keep coming to Lloyd, kissing him and making a fuss. I am filming every minute with my trusty camcorder.

Our weekend was fantastic, but Lloyd has no strength and sleeps two to three hours daily. But we still had a brilliant time.

Sunday is here, and we are making our way back home. First, we will travel to London and stay the night in the same hotel. And then, we will go to Paddington to catch our train back to Newport.

Starlight Charity organised all this. Thanks to them again for such a wonderful time.

Lloyd's tummy is still causing problems, and I am worried about it, so I am taking him to our usual family GP.

I am more worried today because his tummy is large, and there's clear fluid when he breaks wind. Lloyd has a shunt, which they have fitted in his head. The tube from the shunt travels down into his stomach and drains the fluid from his brain. And they know this as CFS fluid.

The CFS disperses into the stomach and then disappears with other body fluids. But I feel the shunt isn't working.

So, I'm taking Lloyd to our doctor to ask if he thinks the shunt is faulty, and if so, how it happened.

Wednesday, 29 August 2001.

We visited our doctor today, and I explained my thoughts about the shunt and asked if my concerns were correct. He replied, "It is not the shunt causing Lloyd's swollen tummy. It's constipation."

I explained Lloyd's loose bowel movements and the clear fluid passing wind. He dismissed this, giving Lloyd lactulose medicine for constipation and said to take it for two weeks.

But I am a mum, and I'm not thrilled about his diagnosis.

It's Monday, 3 September 2001, and our nurse is coming today to place a needle in Lloyd's port-a-cath to flush the line. She will leave it overnight because he has an MRI scan tomorrow to see what the radiotherapy has done to Lloyd's tumour.

Tuesday, 4 September 2001 and today, Lloyd will receive his MRI scan. We now know what to expect because he has had several in the past. They are uncomfortable and noisy, and I feel upset for Lloyd.

A week has passed, and Lloyd is feeling more pain in his tummy. I have received a letter from the oncologist, and he would like to see us on 12 September 2001. I will query Lloyd's tummy problems with the oncologist.

Today, I have been dreading the results of Lloyd's MRI scan. I should be positive, but I have always felt negative about the outcome. And I can't explain why, but because of Lloyd's tumour, I have a horrible feeling that the radiotherapy hasn't worked.

So, as I sat in the doctor's office, he asked the nurse to take Lloyd to the playroom, so I knew the news coming for me would be grave.

The doctor said he was sorry, but the radiotherapy was unsuccessful and further explained that Lloyd only had 6-8 months to live.

These words devastated me, and I went hot all over, and my body shook from head to toe, but I had to stay brave for Lloyd.

They called Lloyd back into the office, but he asked no questions. If he had, I would have told him the truth, not there, at home, my way, but he asked nothing.

As always, he came into the office smiling, so we explained Lloyd's stomach problems to Dr English and my opinion on what I thought was causing it. So he examined Lloyd.

The doctor said I was correct in my assumptions, that the CSF fluid was draining from the brain and into Lloyd's tummy and that there was a blockage, which needed correcting as soon as possible.

He then said we must go to the University Hospital of Wales for an operation, but I could not believe what was happening to my darling Lloyd, and I kept asking what this child did to deserve this.

He is only nine years old, a fantastic, loving little boy who touches the hearts of everyone he meets.

The doctors tell me he has 6-8 months of life left, and straight away, he has to go for another operation.

But what annoyed me most was that I told our GP I thought it was the CSF fluid causing Lloyd's tummy problems, and he said it was constipation.

I am so annoyed about this, and when I have helped my baby through this trauma, I will make an official complaint.

The specialist who fitted Lloyd's shunt is coming this afternoon to speak with us and plan for his operation.

Before he comes, Lloyd requires several tests.

The first test is to clarify that it is CSF fluid in his tummy. So they took us to another room.

They explained what they would do and that they'd insert a long needle, with a syringe, into Lloyd's tummy to draw out some fluid to test.

They will do it without anaesthetic or an injection to deaden the area, so because of the time this will take, Lloyd will be connected to an ultrasound machine, enabling them to see where the needle is going, and then they can draw out the fluid.

When I saw the size of the needle, it worried me, but Lloyd said, "Don't worry, mum, I'm not bothered if they put the needle straight in me; I want to get it over and done with."

They inserted the needle, and Lloyd yelled with a painful cry because it went into his tummy and made a pop sound, so I kept asking, " Why is this happening to my baby? Because this is awful?

The surgeon came to explain what he was going to do.

He will remove Lloyd's shunt from his tummy area and attach a new shunt called a VA shunt, which will enter the jugular vein in his neck and flow through the bloodstream instead of his tummy.

Because they have attached Lloyd's port-a-cath to his jugular vein, they need to remove it, which means an incision in his neck, chest, and tummy.

This operation will take place on Monday, 17 September 2001, and I need to sign papers and okay this operation as there could be complications, but he needs to have this done.

They are doing another test today.

CSF fluid has to come from the shunt in his head, and again, they will not deaden the area, like the tummy area, but they will put a needle in and draw the fluid out.

By now, I am frantic, and it's not fair for my baby to be going through all of this after being told Lloyd only has 6 to 8 months to live.

The surgeon shaved Lloyd's hair around the shunt area with a dry razor and no soap; this was painful for Lloyd.

When he found out they were doing this with the needle, it upset Lloyd, so I calmed him down, pulled him close to my chest, and held his cheek with one hand as the doctor pushed the needle into his head.

Lloyd screamed in pain, and I could see why, because when the doctor removed the needle, he said he didn't have enough fluid, so he put it back in again.

When he did this, the fear and pain I saw on Lloyd's face is something I will never forget because what he went through was excruciating.

Then, to top it all, that evening, they wanted to take blood to test, so I said to take it from Lloyd's port-a-cath. But for their reasons, they said they needed it to come from his wrist.

I didn't want to tell Lloyd this because he had had blood taken from his wrist before, and it is painful, so we talked about it, and after a difficult time persuading him, he agreed.

I love him so much, my brave little soldier. God bless him.

They took some blood from his wrist, and he will have his operation tomorrow, so no eating or drinking for Lloyd, and neither will I. Lloyd needs a good night's rest.

Monday, 17 September 2001, Lloyd is having his operation this morning and says he feels fine, has no fear and wants to get it over and done with.

Lloyd's sitting on a chair with his operating gown on, calm and patient, and I often wonder why he asks no questions and never asks me anything, but I am always ready with an answer.

It's as if he knows what is coming next, as I do; there is something so special between us.

They are coming with the trolley to take Lloyd for the operation, and I'm upset and will not show it, but I always worry he will not wake up after the surgery, every mum's nightmare.

I hold his hand as they administer the anaesthetic, kiss each other, and say sweet dreams, my little darling, and then I do the worst thing ever, leaving him.

Then I wait and wait for the nurse's call, "Lloyd is in recovery, mum." But this time, it seems forever.

At last, I got the call that Lloyd is now in recovery. But he's been in the theatre for five and a half hours, and it is now 6.30 pm, and I can't wait to get to the recovery room.

Thank God Lloyd is okay and responding to the nurse. He gave me one of his gorgeous smiles, but his lips are dry, so I put water on a sponge to dampen them.

He's also had a lot of morphine for the pain and is drowsy; they monitor him for oxygen levels, blood pressure and heart rate.

I pray he will be alright, so I'm not leaving his side, and I will stay awake all night and monitor him.

Lloyd slept all night on Monday and all day and night on Tuesday, and it worries me, but thank the Lord, he is alright.

Today, the nurses look at Lloyd's neck, where the surgeons made the incision.

The nurse removed the bandage, and the sight of the cut upset me.

The cut is about three inches, with seven staples holding it together. It upset me so much that I asked to see the neurosurgeon who operated on Lloyd.

When I spoke to the neurosurgeon, he explained why the incision was long. He said that he had to remove the shunt. So he needed to get to it via Lloyd's neck instead of making another cut on Lloyd's head.

They needed to cut his neck to remove his port-a-cath, so they had to cut longer to access the shunt in his head. There is also an incision in his chest where they had to detach the port-a-cath from Lloyd's chest area.

There is a cut in his tummy from which they drained the fluid. I couldn't believe it when the neurosurgeon told me they had drained six litres of fluid from Lloyd's stomach.

When he arrived at the hospital, Lloyd was nine stone. And after surgery, he was eight stone. No wonder my little darling had so much tummy pain.

What makes me mad is the fact that I was right all along. When I took Lloyd to our GP, I told him the CSF fluids were causing his tummy pain.

So I asked to see the neurosurgeon again and told him I explained to our GP my thoughts about the CSF fluid causing Lloyd's tummy pain, and the GP told me it was constipation.

So, I asked the surgeon about the shunt. And he told me that sometimes, with children and adults, they can go wrong and cause problems.

Then I said, "So why didn't the GP listen to me? Instead of giving Lloyd laxatives?"

The surgeon replied. "Your GP isn't a specialist, and he would have thought the symptoms were those of constipation."

But this was no consolation, and I will complain to the practice manager.

A doctor should listen to us mums when our children are ill. And mums often know more about their child's illness than a GP because of everything they learn and go through.

What has happened to my Lloyd goes to prove it? I'm not letting this drop and need to do something for other mums in my position.

It is a serious misjudgement by a so-called professional, and this caused unnecessary pain and loss of quality time for my baby.

Thursday, 20 September 2001. Lloyd is sitting up today and feeling fine. He wants me to take him around the hospital in his wheelchair. Lloyd spends a lot of time in his wheelchair because of his weakness.

I am taking him to the hospital Concourse. It is a shopping centre at the hospital, and I will buy him some presents. I've bought him some pleasant gifts for when he awakes from his operation, and now I will buy him more.

Lloyd has chosen a beautiful box with Winnie the Pooh and Tigger printed on it. He will put all his recent presents in it.

The nurse came today and said they'll remove Lloyd's staples tomorrow, and then we can go home.

We love our home. When we go away on holiday, we always love returning home. And at Christmas, we never go away. We always love to stay at home.

It's Friday today, and the nurse removes Lloyd's staples. I will hold Lloyd's hand as tight as I can during this.

First, she removed the bandage. I have been dreading the removal of these staples. Because they look awful, and the wound is sore.

Lloyd says. "Hurry, please. Let's get this over and done with."

The nurse, with the staple remover, placed it on the first staple and pulled it. It hurt Lloyd so much when it came out, with still another six to go.

So Lloyd said. "I want to count to three after each one and say now. Then you can pull them out."

He counted to three, and they removed the second staple. Then counted to three for the third. I was now counting along with him while squeezing his hand as tight as possible.

I don't know what was hurting him more.

And finally, they removed all the staples and replaced the bandage with a clean one. They have given Lloyd a certificate of bravery; he now has several of these. He will always be my brave little soldier.

We have been in the hospital for ten days. But before we can go home, Lloyd's specialist wants a word with me. I had a long chat with the specialist, who told me there was a chemotherapy treatment in tablet form. But it's not a cure for Lloyd's tumour, but it may prolong his life expectancy.

They have given Lloyd 6-8 months to live, and this drug may extend this by several more months, but there are side effects, and I think my darling Lloyd has gone through enough in his brief life.

Regarding side effects, we've had experience and know what they are. The doctor admitted that this drug might not even work. I need time to think.

Will I let Lloyd have quality time while he is feeling well? Or will I accept the drug for him so I can have him for maybe another month or two extra in my life?

Deep in my heart, I know it's selfish to think that if Lloyd takes this drug, he will be with me longer.

So my decision is NO!!

I want Lloyd to enjoy what life he has left to the full. And with no side effects from chemotherapy drugs, I will make it very special for him.

He deserves quality time after what he has been through, and God will help us with whatever journey we have remaining. So please, God, help us in our last days.

Lloyd still hasn't asked me questions, although he knows the chemotherapy and radiotherapy treatment has now finished. But still no questions?

If he ever has questions, I owe him to tell him the truth. I hope he never asks me, but if he does, I will tell the truth and be careful about what I say and how I say it.

Lloyd is taking this journey as if they had mapped it out. He doesn't moan or complain and never asks, "Why can't I do that, mum?" When watching other children playing.

Lloyd's courage has amazed us, his family and friends, and everyone else who has met him.

I will give Lloyd 100% of my love, kindness, friendship and quality time during the remainder of his life. And this is my solemn pledge as a mother.

Chapter Ten.

Precious Moments.

Lloyd wanted to go to the Star Inn public house today to see all his friends and play on the fruit machines, as he loves playing them and stays there for ages, putting in money and enjoying the thrill of pressing the buttons; he does it so quickly.

If he wins, I say, "If you're enjoying yourself, darling, put it all back in and have fun."

I love watching him enjoy himself because it's as if he's having a small taste of adulthood. He also enjoys playing pool with the older children and adults.

Lloyd is still sleeping for 2-3 hours a day.

Our time at home is lovely, and we enjoy sitting and playing a card game called Uno.

We also play Draughts, Dominoes, Hangman, Gooey Looey, Connect 4, and Snakes and Ladders, and have many precious moments together, holding hands and giving each other kisses and hugs while making the most of every second we have left together.

Lloyd loves me no matter where we are or who is around, and he desires to show people how he loves me; he is special.

We enjoy watching videos, most of which are funny, and Lloyd loves his PlayStation, so when he is ready for bed, no matter the time of day, I go to bed with him and sleep by his side.

I watch him for hours as he sleeps, until I fall asleep. But I won't leave him because I don't want to miss any time we have left.

So, in the mornings, we go down the stairs, and Lloyd has four pieces of toast cut into soldiers with Marmite; he loves it with a Coca-Cola.

Lloyd is eating more of what he fancies, but not large meals.

If we don't go on a day trip and stay home, Lloyd and I visit our local shops in Maindee, Newport, near where we live.

We go into the big Kwik Save store and buy 24 tins of Cola and loads of goodies, and then we pop over to the pet shop to see the birds and rabbits and then the local Pound Shop for a nose around.

He loves to go out for a walk, albeit in his wheelchair, but he doesn't mind, and on our return from Maindee and the shops, we always go to our local park, five minutes from our house, and Lloyd goes on the swing, and this is our daily routine if we have no trips planned.

Today is 28 September 2001, and we are going to Longleat Safari Park.

When I telephoned them and spoke to the management, I told them we were visiting and explained to them about my special little boy, Lloyd, and how I wanted him to have a splendid time. And they did us proud.

They were brilliant and took us around the park in one of their Jeeps. They would take us as close as possible to the animals and tell us all about them.

We travelled in the Jeep for a good two hours looking around, and then, in the end, a gentleman gave Lloyd a gift of a Longleat book and a cute, cuddly lion toy. Lloyd loved the lion toy and added it to his three hundred teddy bears at home.

So, a massive Thank You to Longleat Safari Park for a memorable day, and I will never forget your kindness and generosity.

We visited the Longleat shop to buy gifts for Lloyd. We purchased another lion similar to the one Longleat gave to Lloyd. The one we got in the shop was a lioness; both had crowns on their heads.

We have taken loads of video footage; we video and photograph everything we do. I consider this important for our memories together.

Monday, 1 October 2001, and off to Alton Towers again today, and this time staying in the Chocolate room in the hotel. We will go to the fair first.

We had a brilliant time at the fair and are now going to our room, and what a room it is.

They opened the door, and Lloyd said, "WOW, this is gorgeous."

There was an enormous chocolate machine on the wall, and when you turned the handle, all the chocolate dropped out.

The room is painted violet and white. And the wardrobe takes after chocolate pieces (not real chocolate). I have arranged for balloons to go in the room and for a message to appear on the TV, which reads. "I Love You, My Darling Lloyd."

We stayed in the Coca-Cola room the last time we travelled to Alton Towers. And in the room was a large Alton Towers teddy bear. Today, there will be two because I bought one and put it on the other bed.

I said, Lloyd, "This teddy on the bed is for you, Lloyd. Love from mum."

Behind our bed is a picture of two glasses of milk pouring over the wall. It looks fab. We are having a fantastic time. This evening we had fun, we went to watch a pirate magician. I have filmed the whole day and night on a camcorder, including many photos.

We are off to the fairground today, and then we are heading back home to Wales.

So, after a lengthy journey, we arrived home, and I sat Alton Bear on our living room floor to remind us of a glorious stay at Alton Towers.

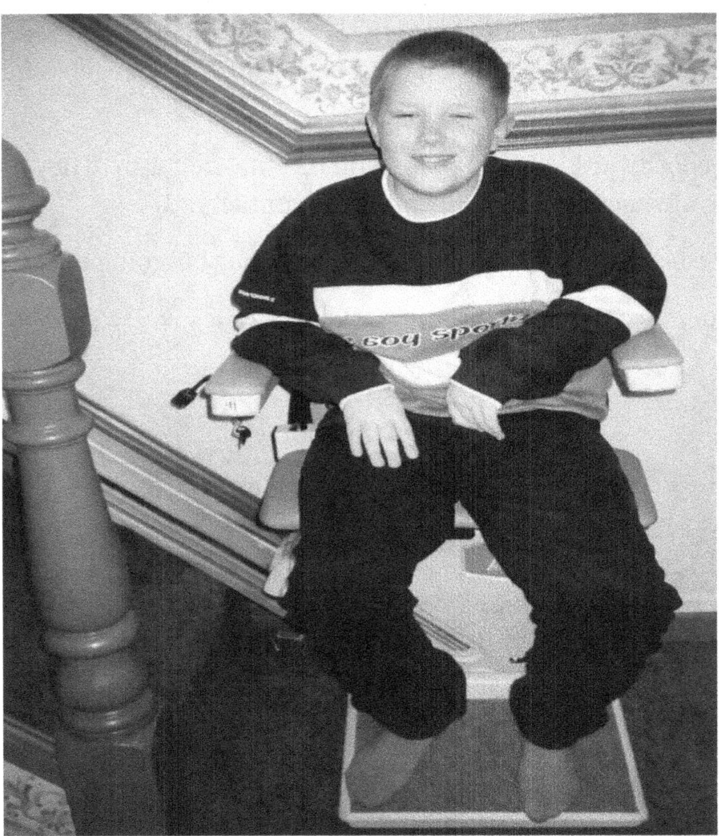

Lloyd on his stairlift.

Today, we are having a stairlift fitted for Lloyd because he is finding it difficult to climb the stairs. A man came to the house to build a platform at the top of the stairs, but I didn't realise he'd be fitting the stairlift too.

I'm not telling Lloyd because he will take his afternoon sleep, so I thought I would surprise him when he wakes up.

The worker was noisy when fitting the stairlift, but didn't wake Lloyd.

Later, when Lloyd woke, I said, "Come and see the platform the man has built on the stairs, Lloyd."

So he came to the stairs to look at the platform and saw that the stairlift was fitted and ready for him to use. He thought it was brilliant. I had sat one of Lloyd's teddy bears on the seat, and when he saw it, he laughed.

I told Lloyd I knew they would fit the lift today, and I kept it a surprise. Lloyd sat on the stairlift and rode it up and down the stairs.

It is so much easier for him now, and we should have had one fitted a long time ago when Lloyd was having his chemotherapy. Better late than never. We have also installed a seat in the bath to make it easier for Lloyd to get in and out because of his loss of strength.

LATCH- the charity at Llandough Hospital is fantastic for us. They have given us an answering machine so the hospital can contact us.

Lloyd sang a song on the answering machine for our outgoing message.

It goes like this.

> "Hello, this is Lloyd,
>
> I'm sorry I'm not home,
>
> But if you leave your name and number,
>
> I promise as soon as I get in, I'll phone."

It is lovely to hear him singing.

Lloyd hasn't attended school since July 2000 and would love to see his friends. I have tried hard to enable Lloyd to visit the school for two hours daily. And to have some normality in his life and be like the other children.

The headteacher, Mr Thomas, has invited us to the school for a talk. Lloyd's last class teacher, Mrs Carter, took him into his old class to look around, but the children there were a year younger.

Lloyd and Mrs Carter were in the classroom for an hour and a half while Mr Thomas and I chatted privately in his office. He agreed to allow us to come to school for an hour and a half in the mornings.

This morning, we are in Mrs Carter's class on the ground floor and have a seat together. They have given Lloyd maths homework to do.

And though he has been out of school for over a year, and despite all the treatment they have given him, he has finished his schoolwork with no help from me.

Lloyd was lent to me by God. So, I will make the rest of his life exceptional with me.

Friday, 5 October 2001, and no school today, except for teacher's training, so we are off to the caravan for the weekend.

This morning, we went swimming. We stayed in the pool for an hour and a half; our skin got wrinkled, but we had a great time.

Later, we will go to Ilfracombe to have fish and chips by the harbour wall. Then we are going to the amusement arcade to win more teddy bears. Lloyd loves it here.

Monday, 8 October 2001. We couldn't go to school this morning as Lloyd is feeling unwell. I contacted the headteacher to explain, and he understood, saying to return when Lloyd feels well enough and not for us to worry.

Tuesday, 9 October 2001. Today, Lloyd feels he wants to go to school, God bless him, and he wants to wear his school uniform. He looks gorgeous in it.

Lloyd has had a fabulous time today, and we spent the morning in the classroom with the year-five children. These were the children Lloyd went through school with from the start of his schooling.

Although Lloyd has missed over a year in school, they will let him stay in the same class with all the children he already knows.

However, he doesn't have to do the same as they do. They are giving him year four work. All the children have been fantastic to Lloyd, and they understand his circumstances.

We have to go to school every day, and Lloyd enjoys it. He likes his teacher.

It worries me because it upsets Lloyd about catching up with the other children's schoolwork. I spoke with his teacher and asked her to reassure Lloyd that he doesn't have to catch up on the lessons and enjoy the work he is doing.

Lloyd seemed better after his teacher had explained the schoolwork to him.

The weekend is here, and Lloyd has a lot of back pain. He slept for two hours this morning, from 11 to 1 o'clock and again this evening from 5 to 7. Despite this, Lloyd still has pain in his back, so we went to bed at 8.30, and I hope he will feel better in the morning.

Lloyd got out of bed and still has a backache. I told Lloyd we should have a day at home from school to rest. But he wants to go.

We went to school for two hours, but it tired Lloyd, and his back was still aching. He also had an itch on his side, which was sore. When I looked, I could see a nasty rash, and I thought it was shingles, so I took Lloyd home and phoned the doctor.

The doctor came to our home and examined Lloyd. He said Lloyd had shingles and prescribed antibiotics for him to take five times a day for seven days. It's so awful.

Why does this keep happening to him? He has been through enough already.

Several days have passed, and Lloyd is feeling okay, but I have noticed his vision is worsening, and he has stopped using his right arm.

22 October 2001. Today we are going to Pontins in Blackpool for a week. It is Lloyd's last day to take the antibiotics, and we are determined to have a splendid time.

We booked into our room after a long journey; the room is fine. We will have our breakfast and evening meals at the restaurant, but Lloyd still isn't eating well, and the smell of food makes him feel sick.

Throughout the week, we will visit Blackpool to win lots of bears and buy gifts for Lloyd. Then at night, we will see the lights.

Today, we went for a ride on a horse and a cart. It was great. We then went to a joke shop and bought some funny things, including a tube that a snake pops out of when you open it.

We went to a fairground in the evening, and I tried hard to win Lloyd a soldier teddy.

To win the soldier teddy, you had to open a card. And if it read 99 when opened, you would win the teddy. Lloyd opened the card, and we were excited because we thought it said 99. When we took it to the man at the stall, he said it was 66. It upset Lloyd and me.

I couldn't see Lloyd crying like that; it broke my heart. The man had made me mad because he had an " I don't give a damn attitude. So I asked if I could buy the soldier, and the man said, "Give me twenty quid, and you can have it."

So I paid him £20 and gave the teddy to Lloyd, and he smiled his gorgeous smile, so it was worth it. I would have paid £100 to see that smile. I never want to see him sad again.

Lloyd sat the teddy on his lap, and we have some great photos and videos of this.

The Sun was shining this morning, so we went for a walk. Lloyd had an orange lollipop, and I had ice cream. I bought a fabulous hat covered in glitter, and we walked along the promenade in the afternoon.

Well. A week has passed already, and we are going home today.

We have forty teddies packed into our car, and the giant soldier bear is in the front passenger seat, wearing a safety belt.

He looks so funny, and the passing motorists are laughing. Lloyd chose our car; we have a disability finance car. It is a mint green Ford Focus saloon, and we love it.

We are now home and looking forward to Lloyd's tenth birthday. I have arranged everything secretly so it will be an enormous surprise for Lloyd.

He knows I always do something fantastic.

Tonight. I've decorated the room with Happy Birthday banners and balloons, and put all his presents on the floor in the living room.

It looks like Christmas. Lloyd deserves everything he gets. I love to make birthdays, Easter and Christmas special occasions for my darling boy.

Wednesday, 31 October 2001. Lloyd's tenth birthday. I can't stop feeling sad, but I must not let it show. It saddens me because this will be his last birthday with us together.

 I wish I didn't feel this way. But I can't help it. I want to make this day as fantastic as I can.

Lloyd woke up this morning at 2:45 to open his presents. We went downstairs, and when Lloyd opened the living room door, his face was a picture of happiness.

Lloyd said, "Oh, thank you, mum, for everything. I love you."

I replied, "And I love you too. You deserve everything you get. You are a brave little soldier."

Lloyd took hours to open all his presents, then went back to bed for a few hours' sleep. I filmed all of Lloyd's birthday morning with the camcorder mounted on a tripod. And this was so we could both be in the birthday video.

This afternoon, I have another surprise for Lloyd. I have a white stretch limousine collecting me, Lloyd, and his friends to take us to the Mega Bowl for his bowling party.

Lloyd could see the limousine parked outside our house, and with a gorgeous smile, he gave me a massive hug. Then kissed me and said thank you, Mum.

We drove around collecting the other children and then headed to Mega Bowl. And after our games, we all went to the Wimpy Bar for food. Lloyd had a Harry Potter birthday cake and blew out the candles after we sang Happy Birthday.

He ate his chicken nuggets and chips, and we gave the other children party bags full of sweets. I organise this every year.

Lloyd had a fantastic time, and it was marvellous to see him enjoying himself after the sadness on his ninth birthday. All he did was lie on my lap because he was ill due to chemotherapy.

But this birthday was fabulous, and Lloyd enjoyed every minute. It makes me happy because everything has turned out so well for him. I will never forget this day for as long as I live. It's brilliant to see Lloyd happy.

The limousine arrived to take us all home, and the limo company gave Lloyd a model of a white limousine. They have got to know him well because we have had several limousine rides. We even had one take us to Llandough Hospital.

We dropped all of Lloyd's friends back at their homes, but I never took Lloyd home because I had another tremendous surprise for him.

As the limousine was getting nearer, he was getting more excited, and this was because we were getting near the Celtic Manor Hotel.

I said, "Surprise, surprise, Lloyd! Happy birthday, darling. We are staying here for two nights; another birthday present."

We pulled up outside the hotel entrance in style. Then the porter, Chris, a friend, was waiting for us, and he opened the limo door.

All our family was waiting there, and they sang Happy Birthday as we exited the limousine.

It was so special for Lloyd. Even our friend Dawn, a manager at the Celtic Manor, dressed up as a witch for Lloyd because it was also Halloween. She came to the hotel on her day off.

Lloyd was overwhelmed, and he thought it was splendid. We went to our room, and they let Lloyd open the door and shouted, WOW!

The room was full of balloons, Happy Birthday banners, and dishes of crisps, sweets, chocolates, party poppers and a gigantic bowl full of water for apple bobbing. There were also many more presents. Lloyd's face was a picture of complete happiness.

When we finished apple bobbing and having fun with our family, friends and the Celtic Manor staff, Lloyd opened the rest of his presents. I then dressed him up in a Halloween costume.

The costume had a SCREAM mask, and when you squeezed it, a tube would cause fake blood to trickle down the face. We went around the hotel, playing Trick or Treat with the staff, and everyone gave him loads of sweets.

Then, the hotel staff handed Lloyd another birthday cake, and they all sang Happy Birthday to him. And this was a special day which will stay in my memory for the rest of my life.

So, later in the evening, everyone went home, and Lloyd and I went to bed. It shattered us after a brilliant day, which he deserved. I had full intentions that this birthday would be ultra special. And so it was.

The following morning, we had an enjoyable time, and in the evening, we went swimming, joined by Lloyd's aunties, in the Celtic Manor pool and the jacuzzi.

Before we went to bed, I told Lloyd it would be fun if we let a balloon go from the tenth floor. So we took a balloon in the lift to the tenth floor, let it go, and then went back down to see if we could spot it in the sky.

 We couldn't, but it was fun looking. Our weekend was fabulous, and we had a fantastic two nights. We also had a brilliant time playing with Lloyd's recent birthday presents.

Monday, 5 November 2001. Back to school today for two hours. Lloyd is enjoying school, and I love going with him.

Tonight is bonfire night, but Lloyd doesn't want to go anywhere, so we stayed home with many sparklers and party poppers instead.

Lloyd didn't feel like lighting the sparklers, so we only popped the party poppers. To make it more fun, we also put up our Christmas decorations. He thought it was a brilliant idea, and we had splendid fun doing it.

Today, we are visiting the local newspaper office here in South Wales, known as the South Wales Argus. I organised it months ago because Lloyd was interested in how they printed the paper.

The staff were pleasant and showed us around the building, including the print room, and gave Lloyd a copy of the latest printed newspaper. They took our photos. We had a fab day.

But today, when Lloyd woke up, he had terrible pain in his left eye. He said it felt as if it was turning around and painful, and this has happened twice before, but the pain doesn't last long.

We went to school, but Lloyd seemed tired. I spoke with him and told him he didn't have to go to school anymore. He said he didn't feel well enough, so I explained to the headteacher, and he understood.

Lloyd's photograph was in the South Wales Argus newspaper today. And they printed a story about our visit to their offices. It pleased Lloyd; he has been in the paper several times now.

It worries me about Lloyd. I can see a huge difference in him, so I am contacting his specialist today to explain how Lloyd feels. They sent a specialist nurse to our home to see Lloyd, and my feelings were right.

Things are happening quicker than I expected. I know my baby, and things are not right. The specialist nurse came to see Lloyd and has planned for us to spend a week at Ty Hafan Children's Hospice, Sully, Vale of Glamorgan.

They told us that if Lloyd doesn't like it, we can come home earlier and don't have to stay there for the entire week.

I explained to Lloyd that Ty Hafan is an exceptional location, a kind of hotel where children who have had treatment can go for a holiday, and there are nurses to look after them.

I made him understand that this place was more of a hotel than a hospital. Lloyd said he would love to go, complained about nothing and said he would try it.

I love him, so I will make it exciting for him. We packed our clothes and toys as if going on a splendid holiday.

Monday, 12 November 2001. We are off to Ty Hafan today for five days; they're closed at weekends. When we arrived at the car park, I looked at the building, and my first impression of it reminded me of an enormous Spanish Villa with beautiful gardens and parks.

At the rear of the building was the sea, with a glorious view, so they welcomed us inside. It is beautiful, new, clean and fashionable.

A nurse stayed with us for the day. The nurses don't wear uniforms to make the children feel more comfortable in their surroundings. She showed us around the building. And all I can say is that it is fantastic. The word I would use is tranquil.

The look on our faces when she showed us the room where we would stay was priceless. It's not a room but more like an apartment of our own at the end of the corridor.

It had an enormous bedroom with two beds for us, so I will pull these together because I love to be near him. There is a living room with loads of furniture and a TV. There's also a bathroom with a shower and towels. A kitchen with a cooker, refrigerator and everything we need. We think it's fabulous.

They required me to fill in a form regarding Lloyd's illness and asked me a painful question. But I understand why.

She asked me if Lloyd becomes very ill (because of his cancer), do I want him to go to the hospital? Or stay in Ty Hafan? I chose for him to stay in Ty Hafan.

Lloyd has spent enough time in the hospital.

They asked me if, in the worst-case scenario, I wanted Lloyd resuscitated.

My answer to this was no.

But if Lloyd wasn't ill and needed resuscitation after an awful accident, then yes. But because of how aggressive his tumour is and knowing they can do nothing for him, I say no.

I felt it would be cruel to bring him back only to be in a worse condition than before. We mums understand these things and would never be selfish.

 And this is hard, but I had to say it, and I believe I am right in my decision. I explained to the nurse that I would never leave Lloyd's side and would attend to his every need. They are granting my wish.

I will do everything for him, including giving him his medication. I have a red emergency button in the room; all the rooms have these, and I only need to press it if I require help.

I feel very safe here with Lloyd because there is always someone qualified at hand.

It worried me today because Lloyd's eyes blacked out for about seven minutes this morning, and he was in complete darkness. He is okay now, but I hope it doesn't happen again.

I pray every night for a miracle for my baby not to go blind.

They have a jacuzzi here. Lloyd loves a jacuzzi. There is also a music room and a sensory room containing beautiful lights.

Everyone here has their meals together in the dining room. They have a fabulous playroom where you can assemble things, such as Christmas cards and calendars. The glitter room has plenty of things to make and do.

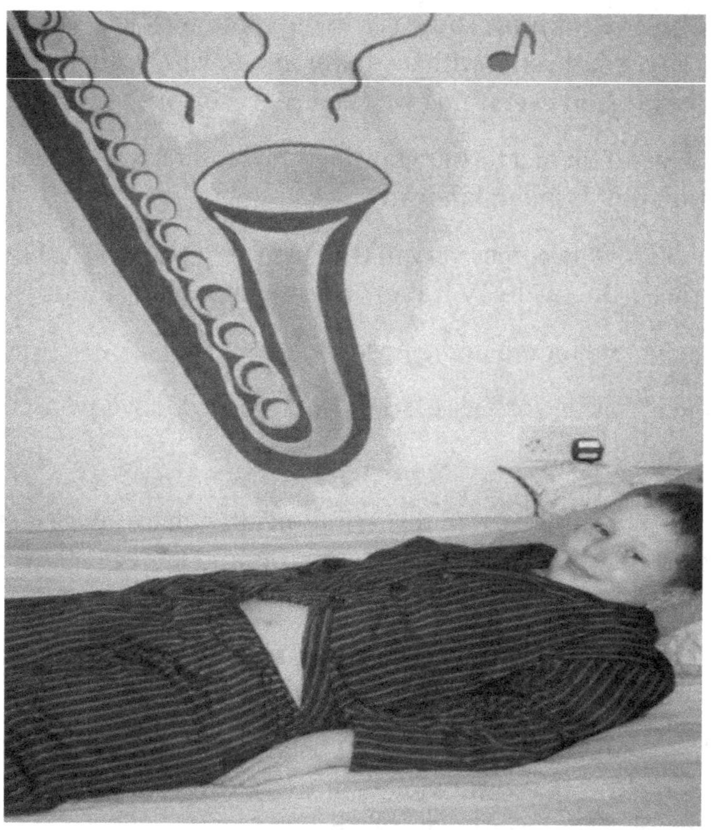

I can't believe it's Friday, and it's time to go home. We've had a fantastic time, and they have invited us to return in December 2001 for another week. Lloyd is looking forward to it.

Lloyd woke up this morning with a painful headache and pain in his right shoulder. And he can no longer use his right arm? I am giving him Medinol (paracetamol) for the pain.

Lloyd is still in pain today, so I am taking him to the GP. The GP gave us Codeine.

Lloyd has taken the Codeine throughout the day, but it isn't making any difference, and it worries me. So if Lloyd isn't feeling any better in the morning, I will take him to Llandough Hospital. And I think he will require regular pain relief.

Lloyd was sick four times throughout the night and again this morning, and he had a headache and shoulder pain. This morning, his eyes looked distant, with small pupils.

I think something is happening, and Lloyd will soon require palliative care.

We went to Llandough Hospital, and they found a bed for him. He was screaming with the pain he was having in his head. And that's not like my Lloyd, so I know something is wrong.

They checked Lloyd over, and it seems I am right. Things are happening, and he needs regular pain relief. He is still sick, and to see him suffer so much breaks my heart.

They gave Lloyd morphine every four hours, and we know it as Oramorph. He must also take ondansetron, an anti-sickness medicine, every eight hours.

I also have antihistamine medicine for Lloyd because the Oramorph can cause itching. I need to wake Lloyd to take it, but he needs rest. I think it's terrible that I keep waking him to take his medicine.

I will check if there is another method of pain relief.

When Lloyd woke up at 6:00, his eyes were blurry again. I hope and pray he doesn't go blind. He wanted to relax in a bath, so I filled the water with plenty of bubbles.

So he sat in his bath lift and fell because he had no control over his body weight. I got him back out of the bath and put him into bed. He is drowsy, and his eyes worry me.

Lloyd hasn't passed solids for several days. So, I believe the morphine is causing this. It concerns me about Lloyd by the minute, so his specialist nurse came to see me today.

I need to discuss things further concerning his pain relief. The nurse is showing me an alternative method of administering Lloyds pain relief. And it's a patch we can put on his arm, which releases the medication every hour. It lasts for three days.

They know the drug as Fentanyl, which is much better for Lloyd, and it pleases me because it is one less medicine he has to take.

But Lloyd never complains when he takes his medicine; he opens his mouth, and I pop it in, even though it tastes awful. I know this because I always have the first spoonful of any alternative medicine he has to take, and I tell him how it is.

I always tell him the truth, and the truth is, they all taste awful. So Lloyd has chewing gum to take away the taste after every spoonful of medicine.

He's had his patch on since 18:00. It's now 20:00, and he still has a lot of pain, so I gave him some Codeine.

They have put Lloyd back on steroids because the tumour is getting more aggressive. He is only taking a five-day course of steroids, and then Lloyd will have a slight break from them, and then he will receive another five-day supply.

He is still taking anti-sickness tablets, and I will not give him more Codeine, but if he still has pain while on the patch, I can offer him Oramorph in between. I must record this so they can work the dosage increase out for each patch.

Friday, 23 November 2001. Lloyd went blind for 15 minutes this morning. It frightened him very much. His sight came back, but his eyes were blurred, and he couldn't make out his surroundings.

Lloyd went to bed this afternoon and slept through the night. He is now sleeping through the day, only waking for his medicine and sips of water. He has eaten nothing since Tuesday.

Lloyd's medication involves him taking Dexamethasone (his steroid), Fentanyl Patch, Oramorph when needed, ondansetron, anti-sickness tablets, and Tegretol medicine, which helps Lloyd to stop having seizures.

The specialist nurse has given me rectal tubes to insert into Lloyd's bottom if he has a seizure. I hope, to God, he doesn't, but I have them in case he does.

The nurse contacted Ty Hafan Children's Hospice because Lloyd's condition had worsened, so they invited us to stay earlier than the planned date of our second visit on 17 December 2001.

I told Lloyd we were going on another break to Ty Hafan, and it pleased him because he loves it there, and he says it's like going on holiday.

Monday, 26 November 2001. Lloyd has been okay, still sleepy, but now cannot speak. He is getting his words muddled up, which frustrates him.

Lloyd can get out of his wheelchair but needs help at all times. If he tries unaided, he will fall, but I am always there for him. I never leave his side, ever.

We walked around the hospice, but now Lloyd feels he needs to lie down and rest.

Today, the Palliative doctor is visiting us at Ty Hafan, so I explained my feelings about Lloyd to the doctor and told him Lloyd was sleeping more than he was awake. He only wakes if I wake him for his medication, and I feel this is a cruel thing to do.

He isn't eating and hasn't passed solids for a week, so the doctor has given me lactulose for Lloyd to help him with his constipation.

Lloyd woke up when the doctor was there and came into the living room to meet him. Lloyd has a considerable amount of pain in his neck.

The doctor touched Lloyd's neck, and it hurt Lloyd a lot. Then, the doctor explained it was nerve pain caused by the tumour. He then gave me more medicine for Lloyd, and Lloyd slept.

I told the doctor I feared my baby was slipping away from me. The doctor said he was sorry to say it, but my feelings were right, and Lloyd was slipping away. He also said it may be a long while, and Lloyd will have good and bad days.

Then the doctor said it amazes him how we deal with everything, and he can see how close we are to each other. I told him that Lloyd and I have unconditional love for each other and will have this love for eternity.

He also said that he sees I am in total control of everything and will always be open with me, and I said that he must tell me the truth no matter what.

I always seem to know everything, even before they tell me anything and sometimes before it happens.

Lloyd woke today at 7:15 and returned to sleep at 7:45. He woke again at 11:45, and then at 11:50, they gave him morphine. He then stayed awake until 16:30.

We went into the jacuzzi to help Lloyd with his pain, but we never started the bubbles. The water is still, and Lloyd loves to sit in the jacuzzi and lean against me. We stay in there for ages, and our skin is withered when we get out.

I had to change Lloyd's pain relief patch on his arm because it had got wet, but that wasn't a problem. After the jacuzzi, Lloyd wanted to go straight back to bed.

Lloyd woke at 5:45 and felt like eating some toast, and this pleased me because he had six pieces of toast with Marmite; I make two at a time.

When he finishes two, I make two more, so it stays nice and warm. He enjoyed it, and it pleased me because Lloyd passed solids, and his tummy felt much better.

Another week has passed, but Lloyd has slept most of the time. And when he has a better day, I will take him somewhere nice.

Lloyd woke at 6:30 and had four pieces of toast and Marmite, a glass of apple and blackcurrant juice. And also a glass of his favourite Coca-Cola.

He went back to sleep at 10:15. When he woke again at 12:15, he felt well, so I took him to the Celtic Manor Hotel to see the Christmas decorations they'd put up inside and outside the hotel.

There was also a model railway at the hotel, and Lloyd thought it was fantastic and liked it a lot. He went to bed at 19:30.

Tomorrow we are going to the garden centre where my brother works to see all the Christmas decorations.

The garden centre was brilliant, and we bought many things for Lloyd. We have had a fabulous weekend and are returning to Ty Hafan the following day for our third time. Lloyd loves it there.

Monday, 3 December 2001. Lloyd woke at 5:00, ate five pieces of toast and Marmite and returned to bed at 6:30. He woke at 8:30, so we left for Ty Hafan and arrived there at 10:15.

Lloyd wanted to go in the jacuzzi, so we did that on our arrival, and he had a pleasant one-hour relaxation. Later, we sat down to lunch with everyone else at Ty Hafan. Lloyd had his favourite chicken nuggets and chips and went to bed at 13:30.

He woke again at 15:30, so we lay on the bed and had an enjoyable chat. Then, he went back to sleep at 18:30 and slept all night.

When I awoke the following day, I found a letter under our apartment door. It was nothing unusual because the nurses always left Lloyd's love letters under the door, but this one was different.

The letter was sent to Ty Hafan by a gentleman we know as Michael; I have met him, and it touched me when I read it.

In it, he wrote that all the people who visit his church were praying for Lloyd, and they had given us a handkerchief (in a plastic bag) they had blessed with holy oil, for me to place it on Lloyd when he is asleep.

It was a beautiful suggestion. Before Lloyd woke, I placed the handkerchief on his head, prayed to God for a miracle, removed it from Lloyd's head and put it under his pillow.

I wrote a thank-you letter to Michael and his friends explaining what I had done.

When they diagnosed Lloyd in 2000, I was able, through a friend, to get some holy water from Lourdes. I placed that upon Lloyd's head and said another prayer for a miracle.

Lloyd woke at 5:00, had toast with Marmite, and returned to bed at 5:45. He woke again at 9:00, watched some of his cartoon videos and then went back to sleep at 12:15. He only eats breakfast and never feels like eating for the rest of the day.

At 14:00, Lloyd woke up, and we went to the jacuzzi. We go to the jacuzzi twice a day now. Lloyd loves it. Later in the day, we went to the art room with the play specialist. And they told me to wait outside the room because they were doing something special for me.

After a short while, Lloyd came out of the playroom with a Christmas card he had made himself. It is full of glitter and has two reindeer on either side. It is another of his most beautiful creations, and I will keep it forever.

We gave each other a big kiss and a hug. Lloyd is feeling tired now.

I have brought several Christmas presents to Ty Hafan. And this is because a few weeks before Christmas, on Wednesday. They are having a Christmas dinner with all the trimmings. So before Lloyd goes to sleep, I want him to open a present. He thinks it's great to open a gift before he goes to sleep. He went to bed at 18:00.

Lloyd woke at 4:30 today and opened his stocking. I want to make every Wednesday a special day, heading to Christmas. So this day will be Christmas Day.

And it's because I feel sad about the proper Christmas Day in December, and I don't know why, but I feel like let's have Christmas now.

So Lloyd opened his stocking and loved everything in it.

He said, "Thanks, mum. I love you."

Then he went into the living room of our apartment and sat by the side of our Christmas tree. Ty Hafan gave us a tree for our apartment, and it looks stunning. Lloyd opened his present, which is a rotating ball. The lights shine on the wall when our room is dark.

It is very colourful, and we know it as a disco ball.

At Ty Hafan, they have a sensory room. It is a room full of colourful lights and has a water mattress. Lloyd loves it in there, so we will make a sensory room in the bedroom of our home with loads of lights and beautiful things.

I won't keep writing about Lloyd's sleeping patterns, but now he is sleeping more often than he's awake.

We have put tinsel around our heads, and I put on a pair of Santa earrings. Lloyd had a Santa badge and a nose which flashed. We put tinsel on his wheelchair, and then off we went for Christmas dinner.

Everyone was there. Lloyd and I pulled out the Christmas crackers and put on our hats and tinsel. He had Coca-Cola in a posh glass, and we had our Christmas dinner. Lloyd only had a little to eat, so I warmed up his favourite peas instead of the Ty Hafan peas because he enjoys soaked peas but could only manage a little.

But being together at a Christmas dinner table was fabulous for both of us.

Today, Lloyd and I are helping make Christmas decorations for the Ty Hafan Hospice. Lloyd is making a glitter soldier, and we are working on a theme: "A Partridge in a Pear Tree." We are enjoying this day. Lloyd is doing a splendid job of making the soldier, and he is looking well.

The play specialist told me Lloyd is brilliant with his hands, and she will put his finished work on the wall. Then, when Christmas is over, he can take it home, and we will put it on our wall.

Lloyd has put his handprint on the wall in Ty Hafan with the other children. And all those who have been there before.

Prince Charles has his handprint amongst them. So Lloyd has put his blue handprint under Prince Charles'. Mine is there, too.

Later that day, when Lloyd woke from his afternoon nap, Ty Hafan Hospice had visitors who arrived in a helicopter. Lloyd and I sat inside the hospice and watched the helicopter land. I have it all on video.

The pilot showed the children around the helicopter, and Lloyd sat inside it at the controls. He was very interested. Later, we went to the jacuzzi. Lloyd needed to take some Oramorph before we went into the jacuzzi, and while we were in the pool, Lloyd's nose became very itchy; the morphine made this happen.

Today is Friday and our last day. Ty Hafan closes at weekends. Lloyd woke up with a pain in his ear and couldn't hear very well. The nurse put some saline in his ear and cotton wool to relieve the pain.

Before we leave for home, the Ty Hafan nurses put on a pantomime for the children and their families. They will do this every Friday until Christmas. When the pantomime ends, Santa gives the children gifts.

We enjoyed the pantomime; it was fabulous and funny.

Then Santa called Lloyd, and Lloyd wanted to talk to Santa. It was only a short distance, and as Lloyd got out of his wheelchair and walked toward Santa, everyone in the room applauded to see him walking.

It was so touching. Santa gave him a present, a beautiful teddy bear we know as Alfie. Lloyd loves him, and when we go home later, we will keep him on the arm of our settee.

Saturday, 8 December 2001. It's our weekend at home, and Lloyd has slept most of the day but has a blocked ear, which causes him pain. I think pressure from the tumour may cause it, or he may need his ear syringed by the doctor.

We will walk to our local shops because Lloyd likes to buy twenty-four cans of Coca-Cola and carry them back home on his lap in his wheelchair. We will also visit the pet shop to see the small animals.

Tonight, we are going to the Celtic Manor Hotel to have another look at their Christmas decorations and to see his friends. The decorations are beautiful, and Lloyd enjoyed himself.

Then, after our visit, the chauffeur brought us back home in Lloyd's favourite car, The Asquith; Lloyd loves the Asquith. We have had a fabulous weekend, and tomorrow, we are returning to Ty Hafan Hospice.

Monday, 10 December 2001. We are back at Ty Hafan, and the doctor came to see Lloyd today and supplied him with some drops for his ear. The dose is five drops four times daily to loosen the pressure in his ear.

Lloyd slept most of the morning and will eat chicken nuggets and chips at lunchtime.

And in the art room, Lloyd is making silver buttons, and we are adding pretty things to them. They have asked Lloyd to play the part of a soldier in Friday's pantomime.

Lloyd's key worker, Karen, whom he adores, is helping Lloyd make a soldier's hat. It is fabulous, tall, and gold, and has a gold chain at the front for his chin. He tried it on, and he looks gorgeous, my brave soldier.

Today, Lloyd can feel acute pain in his shoulder and arm. He doesn't use his arm at all, nor his hand. He is in a lot of pain, so I gave him Oramorph.

We went to the art room, and I helped Lloyd make decorations and beautiful pictures for our home, all made with glitter. We have loads to bring home. They are now calling Lloyd "The Glitter Bug" because he loves pouring glitter over the pictures we have glued together.

Lloyd empties the entire glitter pot. It's fun for him, and then whatever is left over, we put it back in the glitter pot for next time. It's brilliant to see his face when he tips the glitter.

Lloyd feels tired and has no strength, so he wants to go to bed for a rest. He went straight to sleep, and at 2:30, he woke up because he needed to visit the loo. To save him from walking to the toilet, I have brought his urine bottle, which he uses at home.

Lloyd had a pee but no strength, so I tried to lift his legs and help him back into bed, but he fell onto the floor. And I found it difficult to pick him up because I couldn't lift him, so I called the nurses. They came at once and put Lloyd back into bed for me, and he went back to sleep.

Today, Lloyd still has a lot of pain in his arm, so I gave him more Oramorph to ease it. Lloyd is losing the strength in his legs and doesn't seem able to stand any more. He keeps falling over, and I need to hold him up.

Later in the day, we visited the art room, and Lloyd and his key worker, Karen, produced a fabulous Christmas pudding out of glitter. Lloyd made his own Christmas wrapping paper with tags to wrap the glitter presents he had made.

Lloyd woke at 4:00 for a pee, but again, when he put his legs on the floor, he fell, and with the shock of the fall, he wet himself. I called the nurses for help. They came straight away and put Lloyd back into bed. I washed Lloyd down, and he went back off to sleep.

At 9:00, Lloyd woke up, and he had a terrible morning. He had a seizure, which lasted for about two minutes. His legs, arms, and fingers stiffened, and it frightened him.

I spoke to Lloyd, calming him during the seizure until it passed. Fifteen minutes later, it happened again, for about three minutes. Before the seizures begin, Lloyd gets a shivering sensation and a parched mouth and needs loads to drink during these.

The seizures cause Lloyd's speech to become laboured, making it difficult to explain his needs.

Lloyd had his ear syringed this afternoon. It was uncomfortable, but a relief for him to get it done. The doctor would have stopped, but Lloyd said, "You can continue and finish it."

The doctor put Lloyd's dose of Tegretol medicine up for his seizures. Let's hope and pray he has no more seizures because they frighten him.

Friday, 14 December 2001. Lloyd is a soldier today in the Ty Hafan pantomime. He looked gorgeous, as usual, and it was fun for him. I recorded every moment, and it was fun for him to watch himself performing in the pantomime. It was splendid fun. Later, Santa came and gave out presents to the children.

On our return home from Ty Hafan, we stopped at the garden centre and looked around. Lloyd has a thing about garden centres and loves to look around them.

We then went to a McDonald's drive-through for Lloyd's favourite treat: a box of six chicken nuggets with chips. When we arrived home, Lloyd went straight to bed and slept all night.

Today, Lloyd has had steroids again and takes them in a five-day on, five days off pattern, but this time it is only for three days.

He slept most of the day and woke at 17:00 with a lot of pain in both arms and right leg, and this continued to come and go every several seconds. I gave Lloyd an extra dose of Oramorph, and he fell asleep at 19:00.

Today is Sunday, 16 December 2001.

We went to the garden centre, where my brother works, to see Santa. They also had Owls on view. Lloyd loves Owls and had his photo taken holding an Owl, but he wasn't feeling well.

I took him to see Santa, who gave him sweets. Later, we looked around the garden centre, and I bought him a present. We found a brilliant gift for Lloyd: it's an enormous yacht with two teddy bear sailors. It's gorgeous and is now on the windowsill in our bathroom at home.

We then went to the garden centre cafe, and Lloyd had a Coca-Cola and a bag of chocolate balls. I could see he wasn't feeling well, but he said nothing, so we left for home, and Lloyd went to bed.

Monday, 17 December 2001.

And we are returning to Ty Hafan for another five days. We settled into our apartment room, and then Lloyd wanted to go to the art room to make Christmas cards. We made a card for the chef, with chicken nuggets and chips on the front, made with glitter: gold nuggets and yellow chips.

The chef thought it was fantastic and put it on the refrigerator door. After that, we went to the jacuzzi. Lloyd loved it, and we played by passing the ball to each other.

Lloyd's legs are painful this afternoon, so I have given him a dose of Oramorph. I feel that the patch on Lloyd's arm for pain relief should have the dosage increased. I will speak to the doctor when he comes.

This morning, Lloyd woke at 8:00 and had his toast with Marmite. Then we both got ready and went to the art room, and made more Christmas decorations and cards.

Lloyd's arms and legs hurt him, so we returned to our room for him to rest. The doctor saw us this afternoon, and we spoke about Lloyd's pain. So now he is increasing the dosage on his patch from 25 grams to 50 grams.

Later, we went to the jacuzzi and had a lot of fun. Lloyd's favourite nurse, Karen, will start her shift at 21:00, and Lloyd wants to stay awake until she comes.

The other nurses told her that when she started her shift, she had to go straight down to see Lloyd, which she did. They chatted for a while, and then Lloyd went to sleep.

Lloyd woke this morning at 8:30. He fell while getting out of bed, but he managed to get himself up by leaning on a chair by the side of the bed.

It concerns me about his falling.

He had his usual toast and Marmite but had no strength and went to bed at noon. So Ellie, one of his key workers, came to our room and asked Lloyd if he would go to the dining area because Santa and the soldiers were there visiting Ty Hafan.

I woke Lloyd and asked him if he wanted to go, and he said he would. Ellie brought Lloyd a present from Santa in case Lloyd didn't feel well enough to go to the dining area. So Lloyd opened the gift, it's a rugby player teddy bear.

We went to the dining area, and several Welsh Guards were there with a gentleman whom I recognised from a trip to Highgrove, Prince Charles' home and gardens.

I went to speak with him, and he said it saddened him to hear about Lloyd's condition worsening.

He said. "Come into the office. There is someone here who would love to see Lloyd?"

We went into the office, and the other gentleman was the person who had organised the trip to Highgrove. He is a generous man who takes time off from his business to help children who are ill. He said to Lloyd that it was brilliant to see him again.

Then he said, "Look out of the window, Lloyd. Do you see the big red fire engine in the car park?"

Lloyd replied. "Yes, I can."

The man said. "Well, Lloyd. That is my fire engine. I have brought it here for the children to see. Then, after Christmas, I will bring it to your home and take you for a ride. Or, if you are here at Ty Hafan, I will take you from here. I promise you will have a ride in it."

Lloyd was so excited. When they were leaving, Ty Hafan, Santa, and the soldiers got into the fire engine and sounded the siren as they left the car park. It was splendid fun.

It's our last day today, and I took Lloyd on a steam train to Barry Island. He had a present from Santa, and we listened to a storyteller. It was fabulous, but Lloyd wasn't feeling well.

When we arrived home, Lloyd needed to go to bed and sleep. He still sleeps more than he is awake and has not passed solids for over a week, so he's taking lactulose and Co-Danthramer, which is very strong, but this isn't helping either.

This morning, when Lloyd woke, he had a tremendous thirst and drank a lot, but couldn't quench it and was shivering. So he wanted a warm bath; I lowered him into the bath in his bath chair.

He relaxed for a while, but when he wanted to get out of the bath, the bath seat had run out of power because it required an overnight charge to power it up; I tried to get Lloyd out myself, but I couldn't.

The water was getting colder by the minute, and as I was about to phone a friend of mine for help, who lives several doors away, the phone rang.

It was the same friend whom I was about to contact, so I said, "Please come as quickly as you can."

And in a flash, she was there to help me get Lloyd out of the bath; my poor baby was freezing, so I wrapped him with thick towels to keep him warm, and he lay on the bed.

He thought it was funny later when we had calmed down.

Sunday, 23 December 2001.

Today, we went to the cemetery to put flowers on my mum, dad and grandmother's graves, and Lloyd was lying in the car, in the back seat.

When we returned home, our family came for tea and a mince pie. It exhausted Lloyd, and he went to bed. He woke for a little while and then went back to sleep.

Monday, 24 December 2001.

I have planned something for today, it's a splendid surprise for Lloyd.

He woke at 7:30 and opened his letter from Karen and Hayley, who had handed him a pile of letters. Lloyd must open one each day until 2 January.

 That's when Lloyd goes back to Ty Hafan Children's Hospice.

The letters will tell him how wonderful he is and how they look forward to seeing him after the Christmas holidays.

Lloyd's surprise was arriving at 11:00, and as 11:00 approached, I put Lloyd's coat on him and told him we were going out for a walk.

Then, at that very moment, there was a knock on the front door, so we went to the door to answer it, and Lloyd's face was a picture.

There was Santa Claus, all dressed up and looking brilliant, and Lloyd could see his favourite Celtic Manor Hotel car, the Asquith, parked out front; this excited Lloyd, so Santa and I helped him to the car, and in the back was a sack with Christmas presents.

We drove to the Celtic Manor Hotel, and when we approached the main entrance, many of our friends were waiting outside and all dressed up in costumes.

Staff members of the Celtic Manor Hotel, who have become excellent friends, dressed as an elf and a teddy bear and held an enormous box of chocolates.

Lloyd thought it was brilliant because they had even decorated his wheelchair and gave Lloyd many gifts to open from everyone at the Celtic Manor; I also put presents in the sack.

Lloyd loved everything and had a fabulous morning. Lloyd's friend, who dressed as Santa and was the chauffeur, took us home in the Asquith car.

We had a splendid Christmas Eve, and I took plenty of video footage and photos. Lloyd went to bed at 19:00 and was very excited about Christmas Day.

Before we went to bed, we placed a tin of Cola for Santa instead of his usual milk and mince pie and left Rudolph some sweets this year because we forgot to get him a carrot.

Chapter Eleven.

Our Most Special Gift Of All.

Unconditional Love.

25/12/2001. Lloyd woke up this morning at 08:00. It's unusual because his normal waking time on Christmas Day is around 03:00.

Lloyd stood because he wanted to pee, but fell straight to the floor. So we got him back up, but he didn't look well this morning, and his face was flushed.

I passed him his Christmas stockings that I had made for him; three for the bedroom and three for downstairs.

Lloyd loved his stockings full of goodies, but it saddened me because he couldn't move either of his hands or arms, so he asked me to open them for him.

I dressed up for Lloyd to make this Christmas exceptional for a special little boy. So I dressed as Mother Christmas and had tinsel around my head. I opened Lloyd's stockings, and he loved everything and repeated, "Thank you, Mum. I love you."

We went downstairs, which was difficult for him as he had no energy. We entered the room, and there were presents and loads of balloons everywhere. The living room looked like Santa's workshop.

Lloyd smiled, but he wanted to lie on the settee, sleep and open none of his presents. I know now that this is the beginning of the end, and I am devastated.

For this to happen at any time is heartbreaking, but for it to happen today is devastating because all I want is to make Christmas a special day and be happy for Lloyd.

While he slept, I prayed to God and asked for a miracle and for him to let Lloyd enjoy this day, but Lloyd only woke up to be sick. He slept all of Christmas Day.

The night before, I decorated the dinner table with crackers, blowers, and streamers. I made Lloyd his giant cracker, as every year, but this year, I added teddy bears and set them in seats around the dinner table. We had a table that seats six people, and it looked fabulous; even the teddies had Christmas hats on.

Lunchtime arrived, but Lloyd was still asleep, only waking to be sick. The room was still full of unopened presents. I won't open my presents until Lloyd opens his, and we will open the gifts together.

We didn't get to eat our Christmas dinner at the dining table because Lloyd was asleep day and night, and I didn't want to disturb him, so I left him to sleep on the settee. I borrowed my friend's camp bed and slept beside him.

Boxing Day morning, Lloyd had a little toast and Marmite and felt better. About an hour later, he felt ill again and went back to sleep. Lloyd woke at 13:30, so I asked him to open some of his presents. He said yes, but because he had no strength, I had to help him.

Lloyd wants me to open my presents too. I had a beautiful ring from Lloyd, with blue and white gems, and engraved on the side, it says MUM. This ring is very special. Lloyd and I hugged for a long time, declaring our love for each other.

Lloyd slept on and off most of Boxing Day. During his periods of sleep, he would open a present, and he went to bed at 18:00. He wanted to go up because it was more comfortable for him.

Today is 27 December, and Lloyd's best friend, Adam, is visiting for several days. He is more of a brother than a friend. Lloyd has opened a few presents with me today.

I said, "Your presents have never stayed wrapped for such a long time, Lloyd?"

He thought it was fabulous to be opening presents the day after Boxing Day. This afternoon, Lloyd and Adam were playing with Lloyd's Christmas presents. They had fun with the helicopter I bought him, and Lloyd was laughing and having a great time. It was brilliant to see.

He even had a go on the pinball machine he had for Christmas, but he had an awful pain in his shoulder and went to bed at 18:00, so I gave him an extra dose of Oramorph.

Lloyd slept until 10:00 but had an accident and wet the bed and didn't realise he had done this, so I feel he is closing down. And to me, there seem to be signs that he will not be with me for much longer.

I have noticed that Lloyd's urine is black, and his not knowing he has wet the bed is another sign.

Later in the afternoon, two more special people visited him. Lloyd's key workers, Karen and Hayley from Ty Hafan, came to our house. Lloyd thought it was brilliant that they had come to see him.

I spoke with Karen, Lloyd's key worker, about the colour of his urine and his bed-wetting, and she told me I was right in thinking that Lloyd was closing down.

She told me these things happen as time goes on.

When they left, Lloyd wanted to go to bed because he didn't feel well, but a little later, he woke and said he felt like eating a sandwich, which pleased me, so I made him a cheese and pickle sandwich. He only ate a bit of it, but at least it was something.

He went back to bed and then woke again at 19:30 with awful pain in his arms and legs. I gave him a dose of Oramorph and massaged his arms and legs with Lavender oil; he enjoyed me doing that for him.

He slept from 9 pm Saturday and woke at 6 am Sunday. He isn't eating or drinking much any more because he sleeps more than he is awake. I miss him so much because we play together regularly.

Lloyd has slept for two days and has only woken up when I need to give him his medicine (Tegretol for seizures). He is now getting upset because of having to take his medication, so I have decided not to administer more of the laxatives, but he needs to take the other medicine.

Lloyd has now lost total control of his bladder.

All this began on 25 December, 2001.

Monday, 31 December 2001, New Year's Eve. We are having an early New Year's Eve. It's 10:00, and I have given Lloyd a confetti bag. You squeeze the bag, and it bursts, and all the confetti goes everywhere, so I broke a bag of confetti over my head and made him laugh.

We also pulled crackers, said Happy New Year to each other, and gave each other massive hugs and kisses.

Lloyd tried to stand up but couldn't bend his knee because his leg had locked. So he is unable to get on the stairlift: he has to bend his knees because of the wooden grab rail.

So, from today, he will have to sleep downstairs in the living room.

Tuesday, the 1 January 2002. Last night, I could hear the fireworks exploding, and it reminded me of Lloyd and me last year. We were out until 01:00 and had a brilliant time, but this year, all I can do is cry all night and try to come to terms with losing my baby.

I know he is slipping away from me, and I am devastated. I can't bear it, but I will not show my feelings to Lloyd because I promised him. The strength you need is incredible.

How can this be happening? Why my baby? He is a beautiful, loving little boy. I need strength for Lloyd because he has been brave throughout this.

I gave Lloyd his annual New Year's Day gift because he always has one. It is Poppers the Clown, and Lloyd loves it, but is not well enough to play with it.

When I was ten, my grandmother gave me her bible and wrote inside, "To my darling Elaine, from your loving Nan, God bless."

So I wrote inside the bible next to that message. "To my darling Lloyd, from your loving mum, God bless."

I gave it to Lloyd, and he broke his heart crying. I said, "Why are you crying, my darling?"

Lloyd said, "I don't know why I'm crying. I feel sad."

I believe Lloyd knows what is happening to him and that he is going to heaven, but he doesn't want to upset me, so I feel I need to talk to him and explain things, but I want to find the right moment.

Wednesday, the 2 January 2002. Back to Ty Hafan Children's Hospice after the Christmas break. Lloyd woke at 04:00 with severe pain everywhere in his little body, so I gave him a 10ml dose of Oramorph, and he went to sleep.

He still has no food or drink and is finding it more difficult daily to take his medicine. Lloyd woke at 08:00, and then we travelled to Ty Hafan. Lloyd stayed awake during the journey, but he was quiet and withdrawn.

Lloyd was awake for a while when we got to Ty Hafan, but he was in absolute agony, so he had more Oramorph, and we lay on the bed to relax.

He had a lot of pain in his arms and legs, but after a while, he went to sleep and slept the rest of the day and night. He didn't wake until 01:00 this morning and was still in a lot of pain, so he had another 10ml of Oramorph.

Lloyd loves to have a bath, so I thought it would comfort and relax him to have one. There is a large bath at Ty Hafan with a hoist, and I can lift Lloyd out of his wheelchair.

Lloyd said, "I don't want to, Mum."

I replied, "You know me, Lloyd, I have to be cruel to be kind, and I know once you are in the bath, you will enjoy it, so trust me, darling?"

So I called Lloyd's key worker, Karen, and we filled the bath with water and bubbles, then put Lloyd in the hoist. And this saddened me because it was so painful for him to get into it.

The remote control lifted the hoist, and we lowered Lloyd into the bath. Once in, he said, "Thanks, mum. This bath feels fabulous."

I replied, "Well, Lloyd, I knew you would enjoy it."

He squirted us with a fish-shaped water gun, so I got my camcorder and filmed him.

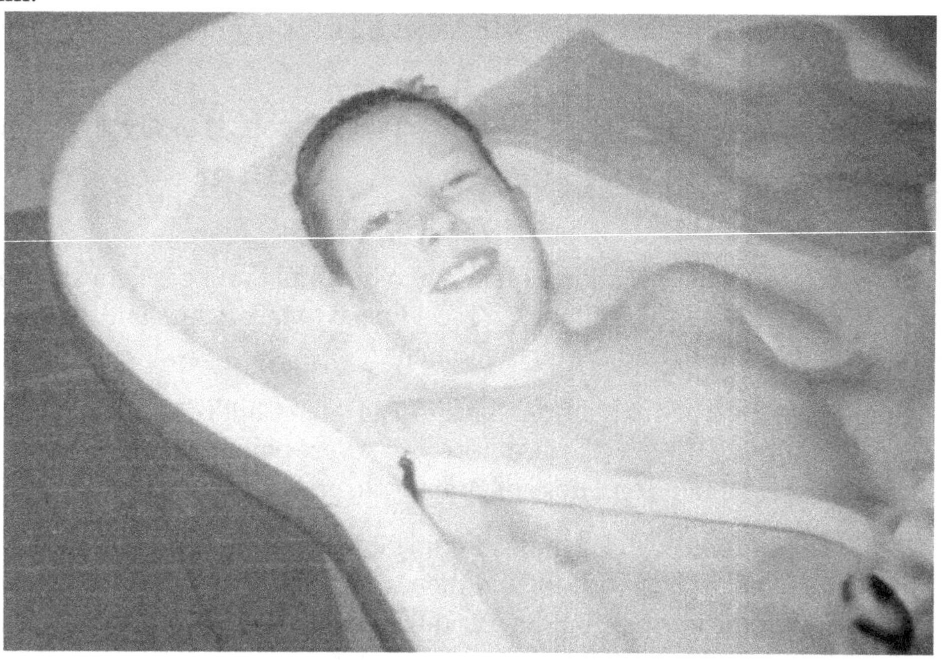

Karen and I helped get Lloyd out of the bath with the hoist, but he was in pain and had a red rash all over his body. The doctor came to the hospice to see Lloyd and said there was nothing to worry about because it was only a heat rash.

I put a dressing gown on Lloyd, and he said, "Please, Mum, take me back to our room. I need to lie down. I'm hurting all over."

So we lay on the bed and listened to Diana Ross' music. Lloyd said she had a sweet voice and went to sleep all night until 08:30.

This morning, Friday, the 4 January 2002. We left Ty Hafan by 10:30, and I had arranged a limousine as a surprise for Lloyd to return home. I didn't want to take him home in an ambulance, and Lloyd wasn't well enough to sit in a standard car.

So I thought he could lie down in the limousine and have more comfort.

Lloyd's wheelchair is no longer comfortable, so Karen has brought a look-alike armchair on wheels; he loves it.

He is even in pain when I put his coat on him; he is in absolute agony. Oh God, why is this happening to my baby boy? The doctor has now put Lloyd's pain relief patch up from 50g to 75g. One nurse came to our room and said, "Lloyd, your lift home is here."

So we went to the entrance, and a man came in the front door and said, "Taxi for Lloyd Pike."

We went outside, and Lloyd's favourite white stretch limousine was parked there. A beautiful smile beamed across his face when he saw it.

The nurses tried to lay him down in the back of the limousine, but Lloyd was in agony. I wish Ty Hafan could open on the weekends so Lloyd and the other children wouldn't have the pain of being moved.

If only Ty Hafan could get more money from somewhere.

It is a charitable hospice that requires one million pounds a year to stay open.

What annoys me, and thousands of others, is the amount of money certain groups of people, such as footballers, are paid a week. And if they each donated a fraction of what they earned, places like Ty Hafan could stay open over the weekend.

Lloyd was in a lot of pain while travelling home and had difficulty getting out of the limousine. The previous night, I telephoned my partner, Gareth, and asked him to get a single bed from his father's house and put it in our living room so Lloyd didn't have to go upstairs.

I thought this would surprise Lloyd when he saw the bed in the living room, but he couldn't see very well and didn't see the bed, and all he could do was say, "I need to lie down," as he was in so much pain.

Lloyd finds it more difficult to speak and gets his words mixed up because of his tumour.

I said, "Look over here, Lloyd. There is a bed down here for you, so you don't have to go upstairs." He tried to smile and lie on the bed. So I lay on a camp bed by his side and played Diana Ross' music for a while. And then we put on the Beach Boys.

He told me he would rather listen to the lady singing, so we put Diana Ross back on. All Lloyd could do was stare at me and find it difficult to speak, so we just lay there face to face, looking at each other. I don't want to leave him.

Lloyd went to sleep at 16:00 and slept all night. I stayed awake watching him because he was making a clicking noise with his tongue on the roof of his mouth and had been doing this for about three weeks.

The doctor said this was a sign of him having seizures, but tonight was different. It was louder and more constant. It worried me.

When we were leaving Ty Hafan, I told Karen I felt I would not have Lloyd in my life for much longer, and I asked for her thoughts. She said, "I believe your feelings are correct."

She also said I seemed to know what was happening with Lloyd. I'm a mum, and I feel what my baby is feeling. I can't go to sleep. It worries me that something will happen, and I don't want my Lloyd to be alone.

Because this is the saddest time of my life, seeing my baby slipping away. When anything happens, I know I will never be the same person again for as long as I live.

I feel like I'm slipping away with my Lloyd, and I wish we could go together, but it doesn't work that way.

Saturday, the 5 January 2002. At 02:00, Lloyd breathed with a loud crackling sound as if his throat was full of phlegm, and I thought Lloyd was going.

When my mum passed away from cancer just before she passed, she had the same breathing noises. It is a terrible way of putting it, but we know this sound as the "death rattle."

As Lloyd was sleeping, I held his hand and wondered whether I should phone his specialist nurse or hug him close to me. I hugged Lloyd tight, then, at 04:30, I called his nurse. But when I phoned, her answering machine was on, so I left an urgent message: it's Lloyd Pike's mum, and I need you to see him.

Then, at 06:00, I received a phone call and explained Lloyd's breathing, but she said she couldn't attend to us until 09:00.

When she arrived, she looked at Lloyd and knew what was happening. I told her that there was no way Lloyd could take his medicine by mouth and that he had slept since 16:00 the previous day.

He didn't seem to be awake at any time of the day or night, and I told her I thought Lloyd was going into a coma. The nurse telephoned the specialist doctor, and they planned to put a syringe driver into Lloyd's arm.

A syringe driver is a small battery-powered machine that contains the medication. A plunger moves and releases the medicine through a tube into Lloyd's bloodstream via a needle in his arm.

I wanted to put Ametop deadening cream on his arm first; I didn't want him to feel the needle going in—he has been through enough pain in his brief life, and I have promised myself that he will not suffer any more.

Lloyd no longer needs the patches on his arm because he receives 80mg of diamorphine through the syringe driver. I am also refusing to let Lloyd take the medicine carbamazepine.

We also know this medicine as Tegretol, which they use to treat seizures.

Lloyd is also having 2.5mg of Midazolam administered through the syringe driver. I am not allowing him to have the seizure medicine, and that's because the nurse said he would have to take it by mouth. After all, they can't give it via the syringe driver with the other medicine.

I said, " Fair enough. If Lloyd needs the medication carbamazepine, I will give it to him via his rectum. The nurse phoned to ask if this would be possible. The specialist doctor said this was possible, so the nurse went to Llandough Hospital in Penarth to get some.

After the nurse fitted the syringe driver, I explained to Lloyd what was happening and how the syringe driver would help him take his medicine.

He could hear what I was saying because he opened his eyes to say, yes, Mum, that's okay. But he isn't talking.

The syringe driver is far better for Lloyd because it adds pain relief when needed. The specialist nurse is organising the community nurses to call our house this evening to check everything is alright and help me with anything I need.

Lloyd has slept all afternoon. He opened his eyes once, and it looked like he was staring at our Christmas tree. He then lifted his arm, pointed his finger to the right-hand corner of the living room, and tried hard to say something.

It wasn't clear what he was saying, and it broke my heart because I couldn't understand him. At first, I thought he was pointing to the Christmas tree, but then I realised he had seen something special. He then went back to sleep.

Later that evening, the community nurses came to our home. There were two of them. Lloyd had wet the bed, so they helped me change the bedsheets, and I washed Lloyd all over.

When I finished washing him, I put a clean T-shirt on him and laid him back on the bed, then he put his arm around my neck and gave me a beautiful hug. I will remember that hug because he put all his strength (what little he had) into that hug. And I will never forget it as long as I live.

It touched the community nurses emotionally to see this because it was beautiful to witness.

I had to give Lloyd his carbamazepine tonight via his rectum, so the nurses watched me and checked I was doing it correctly. The nurses would have done it, but I want to do it for Lloyd.

I moved him onto his side, and it went better than I thought. I'm sure Lloyd felt nothing, and this pleased me because I needed to administer it once in the morning and once at night: 125mg twice daily.

Lloyd had a comfortable night, but lately he has had pain every 15 minutes. To comfort him, we are adding an extra 7.5mg of diamorphine. The nurses believe it isn't pain, and Lloyd tries to cough but finds it difficult.

We settled Lloyd for the rest of the day. We had a lot of visitors to see Lloyd, but I only allowed two people at a time, and they had to be quiet.

Lloyd stayed asleep all evening, and while I was watching his breathing, I had to decide whether to take him back to Ty Hafan on Monday or for him to stay at home.

And I, for my reasons, want Lloyd to be at home when he goes to heaven, but then I thought Lloyd would wish to go to Ty Hafan. I thought about it all night and remembered Karen's words to Lloyd on Friday.

"See you on Monday, Lloyd."

And I know if Lloyd is well enough to decide, he would want to go to Ty Hafan. So we will go to Ty Hafan for Lloyd.

Monday, the 7 January 2002. They have organised an ambulance to take us to Ty Hafan. The nurse called in to change Lloyd's syringe driver, and she put a Hyacinth patch on Lloyd's neck to help with his rattling breathing.

The patch dries up the saliva in the back of the throat and lasts up to 72 hours.

Then the ambulance arrived, and they didn't think they could get the stretcher into the living room.

I said, "Yes, you will, even if you have to knock the stair bannister down. Please try to get the stretcher in the room."

So they did this. There was no way I was going to allow them to put Lloyd in a chair. No way. When they lifted Lloyd with the sheet to put him on the stretcher, he screamed in pain, and this was when I believed I was doing the correct thing by taking him to Ty Hafan. But everything is starting to confuse me.

When we got in the ambulance, the paramedic said, "You must sit in this seat with the seat belt on."

I refused to sit there because I wanted to sit on the floor by Lloyd's side and hold his hand. Nobody will tell me what to do when it comes to my Lloyd, so I sat on the floor of the ambulance by his side and held my baby's hand.

Lloyd is distressed and has an alarmed look on his face. I thought he was in pain, but the paramedic said that the morphine and the travelling were disorientating him.

On our way to Ty Hafan, and again, Lloyd lifted his arm and pointed to the right-hand corner of the ambulance. He tried to say something, but I couldn't understand what he was saying. After Lloyd had pointed to the corner of the ambulance, the paramedic asked me for Lloyd's records, so I told him they were in Ty Hafan Hospice.

I believe the paramedic thought Lloyd was passing away, and he wanted to see his records to find out my wishes regarding Lloyd's resuscitation.

I also feel he didn't want to ask me, in case it upset me. He could have asked me because I knew more than he could imagine. If he had asked me if I wanted Lloyd resuscitated? I would have said NO.

The ambulance ride was traumatic for Lloyd because it was bumpy and noisy, and it disoriented him. When we approached the entrance doors to Ty Hafan, Karen was waiting for us outside.

She looked upset and knew how much Lloyd had deteriorated over the weekend. Karen said we'll do whatever we can to make Lloyd's last few days as pleasant as possible, and for Lloyd and me to be together.

We settled Lloyd into bed, and Karen talked to him. The doctors say that if you are in a coma, you can still hear what people are saying. So Karen stayed and chatted away with Lloyd. And this is what's special about Ty Hafan.

The nurses act as if everything is okay and do their business as usual with Lloyd, laughing and joking around him. We are all around him because I don't want him alone for a second. I only leave his side to go to the toilet while a nurse monitors him.

One nurse had fits of laughter when I asked if I could have a bedpan so I didn't have to leave the room.

Later, I went to the toilet, but the nurse wasn't in the room. And when I was in there, I heard Lloyd call out, "MAM!" I rushed back to the room because I thought something awful was happening.

It worried me because Lloyd was in a coma and not speaking, but I knew he had called me. When I got to him, he lifted his arm and pointed to the right-hand corner of the room again. It was unbelievable, Lloyd called me like that.

He may have seen the spirit of my mum or somebody else who has passed over calling him to heaven. Or it could have been many other things, such as an out-of-body experience. I don't know, and it's more than probable I will never know.

We played Diana Ross's music for Lloyd with many more of his favourite songs. One was the Hamster song, where they swear at the end. It is funny and makes Lloyd laugh, but not today, not at this sad time.

We also put on a disco light in the room, with many coloured lights moving around. I played with a Donald Duck puppet and did the voice, and it used to make Lloyd laugh, but not today.

I am lying by Lloyd's side, and his breathing upsets me. I kiss him and tell him how much I love him. The nurses have given us a different bed for Lloyd. It's an air bed, and it ripples to stop bedsores.

And the thought of Lloyd moving again upsets me, but it's best for him. When they moved him from the bed to put the air mattress on, Lloyd was in a lot of pain, and it upset me.

He also had an accident and wet the bed, and when we were changing and washing him down, I noticed he had a red rash on his poor bum, so I put some Vaseline on him.

It's getting late, and so I will cuddle into Lloyd, but I can't go to sleep. I won't sleep because I want to watch my Lloyd through the night.

Tuesday, the 8 January 2002. Last night, Lloyd's breathing had worsened, and this morning, it seemed as if he was going. I have an awful feeling it will be tomorrow at the latest.

I always seem to know it's as if I have got second sight. I don't enjoy feeling this way, but everything I have been thinking and feeling during Lloyd's illness has been correct.

I want Lloyd's father and my partner Gareth to be here because I know Lloyd would desire that. The nurses contacted them, and they both came straight away.

Another of Lloyd's favourite nurses has come into the room to be with Lloyd. She is a lovely Irish girl we know as Susan. Lloyd could never understand her, but he liked her a lot. So do I. They are all fantastic people.

They gave Lloyd money when he was well, and out of the goodness of his heart, he gave Ty Hafan £50. They used the money to buy a bookcase shaped like an enormous red rocket, and it reached from floor to ceiling.

Anyway, there was a lot of noise outside the room. It turned out to be the nurses bringing the rocket bookcase down to put it in Lloyd's room with him because he had never seen it. So I explained to Lloyd what the noise was.

I said, "This is the rocket you bought for Ty Hafan Lloyd, and the nurses are putting it in your room."

To this day, I wish he could have seen it.

I feel Lloyd is struggling with his breathing because when his dad and I hold his hands, and Lloyd breathes in, it is difficult for him, and he squeezes my hand.

When I looked at Lloyd's dad, he said, "Did Lloyd just squeeze your hand?"

I replied, "Yes, he did."

I was alarmed because I thought he was in pain, but the nurses reassured me and said he wasn't in pain. It was his body's reaction to his breathing. My partner sat at the bottom of the bed and noticed Lloyd's difficulty with his breathing.

After a while, the squeezing stopped, but Lloyd's breathing remained the same: it was heavy with a loud crackle. It upset me to hear him breathing like this; it was as if he was in a lot of pain. But the nurses said he was not in pain.

Everyone has been so fantastic to us, looking after us, and I have permitted my family to visit Lloyd tonight, two at a time. It saddens me so much about tomorrow.

They all came to see Lloyd, and everybody was upset because they all loved Lloyd, and anyone who ever met him loved him.

As the evening and night proceeded, my partner and Lloyd's dad managed to get some sleep. I didn't want to go to sleep, but at 05:00, my eyes closed. And so I threw a pillow at Lloyd's dad and told him to get a nurse to sit with me.

I did this so if I fell asleep, the nurse could nudge me to keep me awake. The nurse came into the room and told me to cuddle in with Lloyd and go to sleep, and if his breathing changed, she'd wake me.

I cuddled into Lloyd at 05:20, and he looked like a gorgeous little angel; I slept with him until 07:15.

On Wednesday, 9 January 2002, when I woke, Lloyd still looked like a gorgeous little angel. This morning, something came over me, and I felt pragmatic; I was letting Lloyd go to heaven.

I have always felt that a child waits for their mum to permit them to do something. For Instance: "Yes, Lloyd, you can go swimming. Or, no Lloyd, no swimming tonight."

So you tell your children what to do. And I felt today I would tell Lloyd he had my permission to go to heaven. But first, I want to make everything extra special for Lloyd.

We opened the blinds and put Freesia flowers in the window. I always kept Freesias because I would pick one and keep brushing it past Lloyd's nose to make the unpleasant smell of his breathing better for him.

I changed Lloyd's bedding, washed him down, gave him a clean T-shirt and massaged his hands, legs and feet with Lavender oil. Then I told him a story of Caitlin and the Kite. It is about a baby girl going to heaven.

I then read him something I had written to Ty Hafan to put in Lloyd's unique bed (coffin), but I read it to him today.

Several of the care team came to see Lloyd, and later, when I was ready, I wanted the nurses to help me lie by Lloyd's side.

I put one hand on his face and held his tiny hand. His dad lay on the other side of the bed, and my partner sat at the foot of the bed. These were my wishes. I was bossy. The nurses went to the other room and waited.

Then I told the nurses that my plan was for us all to go to sleep, and if they heard a change in Lloyd's breathing, please come and wake me. The nurses had an intercom in their room, which connected to our bedroom.

As I lay holding Lloyd, 10:30 came, and I said to Lloyd, "Mum, Dad, and Gareth are all having a short sleep together."

Then I said, "Lloyd, I want to say something to you. Mum is permitting you, Lloyd, to go to heaven with Nanny and bampy. So don't worry about mummy, I will be okay. And when it's time for me to go to heaven, we will be together again, forever and eternally."

Lloyd understands heaven. He has always known that my mum and dad are both there. I also believe Lloyd knew about him going to heaven, and I think Lloyd has been holding on and worrying because he doesn't want to leave me alone.

Our love for each other is unconditional, but I had to tell him he has my permission to go. These words are the most difficult I have ever had to say, especially to my baby, but I feel it was the correct thing to do.

When I said these words to my baby, he had two tears drip down his little face. I wiped them away, kissed him, and said, "We will always be together in my heart. I love you so much, Lloyd."

Then we went to sleep, but my partner stayed awake. I was sleeping, off and on, but I kept watching Lloyd, telling him I loved him while touching his hair.

I said, "Mummy loves Lloyd, and I know Lloyd loves mummy too." At this moment, I must have had my eyes closed because I opened my eyes at 12:10 and looked at Lloyd. And I knew straight away that he was going.

He had mucus coming from his nose and mouth, and his breathing had changed. My partner Gareth passed me a tissue to wipe Lloyd's mouth, and I asked him to tell the nurses that Lloyd was going.

He went to tell the nurses, and they said, "Yes, we know. We heard Elaine, so we are turning off the intercom for your privacy. You know where we are if you need us?"

We then woke Lloyd's dad and explained that Lloyd was going, so Dad held one hand, and I held the other. Gareth stayed, and all we could do now was wait.

I was hugging and kissing Lloyd. It is the saddest time of my life. I held my baby when I brought him into the world, and now I am holding him as he's leaving it. I kept kissing him on the cheek, telling him I love him. Then, after a short while, Lloyd took his last breath.

Then I placed my ear to his chest and heard his last heartbeat. Lloyd's heartbeat will always beat together with mine. Then I kissed him over every single part of his body. It's something I needed to do.

I had my time alone with Lloyd until the doctor came to register his death.

Lloyd Michael Pike passed away at 12:20 on Wednesday, the 9 January 2002, at the tender early age of 10 years. I will always love you, my darling Lloyd.

Later, they moved Lloyd off the air bed and put him onto a standard mattress. The room had to be freezing, and Ty Hafan had air conditioning. I am still adamant that I am not leaving my baby's side.

Catherine, who has been with us all along, told me that Lloyd needs to go to the funeral director's, but straight away, I said no.

So Ty Hafan let us stay there for the night, but I have to allow Lloyd to go to the funeral directors in the morning. And tonight, I had to sleep with Lloyd, so I put on two fleece tops and three continental quilts. The room had to stay cold. I held Lloyd's hand all night and kept kissing him.

This morning, it was time for the funeral directors to come. Karen and Susan, Lloyd's nurses, asked me to leave the room because they needed to put Lloyd on a special trolley. It was difficult for me, but I vacated the room.

Last night, Lloyd was lying on the bed with his dolphin pillow and dolphin quilt over him, and sprinkled on the cover were glitter and sequins because they called Lloyd the glitter bug.

Throughout last night, I listened to Lloyd's favourite sound.

We have a machine that plays the sound of a stream and birds whistling. Lloyd looked so peaceful. No pain, no more medication.

But WHY? And I kept saying to myself, WHY?

Karen and Susan have got Lloyd ready for the funeral director. They brought Lloyd out of the room, and all I could see was a blanket covering his body and face, which upset me. But the blanket covering his face was a special one.

It was white, with red and blue stars, and in the corner it said "Coca-Cola."

Lloyd loved Coca-Cola, but because of the stars, and as I cried, I said, Lloyd looked like a soldier. It was like in America when a soldier gets the stars and stripes flag put over them. I said, "Lloyd is a brave soldier."

The funeral director told Karen and Susan it was like coming to collect a brave soldier. Then he wheeled Lloyd out and put him into the private ambulance. It was dreadful seeing my baby leave Ty Hafan without me.

Lloyd's dad and I had to make several arrangements, and then we said our goodbyes, thanked the staff of Ty Hafan and set off home. It was unbearable going home without Lloyd.

When I got home, Lloyd's bed was still in the living room. I had made previous arrangements with the funeral directors and told them I wanted Lloyd back home as soon as possible and to put him into his bed at our home.

I didn't want Lloyd staying at the funeral director's because I needed him home with me. I have to keep the house cold, with all the windows open. Not long after I arrived home, they came with my Lloyd.

They had dressed him in his favourite clothes: his Nike trainers, white trousers, a T-shirt, and a white Nike jacket. Even his underpants and socks are Nike.

I then placed his dolphin quilt cover over him and sprinkled it with glitter. He looks like an angel. Then I put his teddies around him, and I will sleep by his side tonight and hold his hand. I read Lloyd a story and talked to him for a long time.

Dad and Gareth, my partner, are still here. And it's nice for us all to be here together. I have placed Freesias on Lloyd's chest as this flower will always be unique to me. Lloyd is wearing his necklace, bracelet, and earrings.

Our family and friends came to see Lloyd and to say their goodbyes to this special little boy.

Friday, the 11 January 2002. We are receiving loads of beautiful cards and flowers. Also, Lloyd is in the South Wales Argus, and I know he would have been proud. He has been in the paper several times and thought it was great, but I wish it had been under better circumstances.

They have put my and Lloyd's favourite picture of him on the front page of the local newspaper, saying that he has passed away and where his funeral will be held on the following Thursday. It was heartbreaking for hundreds of us because everyone loved him very much.

We stayed with Lloyd again today, Saturday. I can't stop holding his hand and kissing his beautiful face. We have decided that tomorrow, Sunday, we will have the church curate over to plan for Lloyd's funeral. We will also ask him to pray and cover Lloyd's face with his dolphin cover.

The curate came to the house and did what we asked. He said a beautiful prayer, and I covered Lloyd's face. I still slept by his side all night and held his hand. I also lifted the cover from his face and kissed him.

He is still, and will always remain, my special baby boy.

Sunday has passed, and here we are on Monday already. It upset me about today because they are bringing Lloyd's coffin, or as I call it, Lloyd's special bed.

It is white with brass handles and a brass nameplate on the front. They have arrived with Lloyd's unique bed, and they will put Lloyd into it.

But before they covered his face, I asked them to put his white Nike cap on. Dad and I entered the room and placed a gold folder inside Lloyd's coffin that I had made. It contains photographs of everyone, a colouring from his little step-brother, and Lloyd's special teddies, including the one he had when he was one year old.

I didn't want to part with it, but I wanted Lloyd to take it with him. I have another of his teddies for me to cuddle. We put many beautiful things in with him, including the bible I gave him.

It was then time to put the lid on the coffin. I was anxious about this, so we kissed Lloyd on his forehead, covered his face and said, "We love you."

When they put the lid on the coffin, I put his famous picture on top of it. I will still sleep by his side, in his bed tonight, while looking at his photo and kissing it.

It is breaking my heart because I can no longer hold his hand.

Tuesday. Today, we received hundreds of cards and flowers and have many visitors. My partner has been fabulous and is making tea for everyone.

Another sad and Lonely day and night have gone; It is devastating to me. Wednesday, one week has passed since Lloyd's passing, and it's his funeral tomorrow. I have planned Lloyd's funeral to be beautiful because he deserves the best.

He has always had fantastic birthdays, Easter and Christmases, and his funeral will be beautiful. I have had helium balloons delivered today for tomorrow, and all the floral tributes will come in the morning.

Lloyd will have his name in flowers: LLOYD, from Mum and Dad, and a massive teddy from Mum, Gareth and his son Adam, Lloyd's extra special friend. There will also be a pearly gates arch to heaven from my partner, Gareth and me. An angel from Dad and his wife, and another teddy from his step-brothers. And many, many more.

It worries me about tomorrow because Lloyd is leaving our home, and I find it unbearable. I feel I want to go with him, but it's natural for anybody to feel this way after losing their baby.

Lloyd fought so hard for his life, and he suffered doing so.

So, this is my suffering, and I need to fight for the rest of my life, although I have powerful feelings of not wanting to be here without Lloyd. I had a brave little soldier, so it's my turn for bravery.

I had an exceptional teacher because Lloyd has taught me so much about life and many other things. Lloyd will always be my darling little angel. I have asked God to give me as much strength as possible for tomorrow.

Thursday, the 17 January 2002. On the sides of Lloyd's unique bed, I have hung little white angel teddies to the six brass handles.

Yesterday, because it was one week since Lloyd had passed away, I took a helium balloon and let it go up into the sky at 12:20, the time Lloyd passed away.

It flew higher and higher until it disappeared. Lloyd and I did the same thing once when we let a balloon go and watched it fly until it disappeared. Lloyd enjoyed doing that.

Our family and friends are arriving, but it upsets me because my Lloyd is leaving our home. But I am adamant I will not cry. I want this day to be beautiful for Lloyd. The funeral cars have arrived, and my heart is pounding so hard I can hear it in my ears.

I say it's Lloyd's and my heart beating together, but the reason is stress. I am shaking from head to toe. But I will have to be brave, just like Lloyd. Before we go, I will have one last moment alone with Lloyd in our home.

It overwhelmed me when I went outside the house to see the cars. We had one car for Lloyd with flowers and another full of flowers.

There was a limousine-shaped floral tribute, loads of teddies, angels, an owl (Lloyd loves owls), a butterfly, a pool table and a giant star from his favourite pub, The Star Inn.

The floral tributes were so many that they required an extra car for those alone.

The coffin bearers for Lloyd's special bed are me, my partner Gareth, Lloyd's dad, my brother, my nephew and Lloyd's friend Chris, representing the Celtic Manor Hotel.

I brought my Lloyd into the world, and I needed to take him out to go to his next life. Remember, you never die; you cross over.

Lloyd's special bed was in the hearse, and Lloyd's police officer friend, Boyd, was in his police car, wearing his full uniform out of respect for his little friend,

Lloyd.

Boyd drove his police car in front of the hearse and led the way to the church through the traffic with his blue lights flashing.

The Limousine company sent the white stretch limo we always used for Lloyd to transport all of Lloyd's friends to the church and the cemetery. His favourite car, the Asquith, was also there, along with the staff of the Celtic Manor Hotel.

As we left our home, the funeral director had a photo of Lloyd (the one at the start of this book). I call it his famous photo.

The funeral director carried Lloyd's photo in front of the hearse for everyone to see. People and neighbours around the area stood outside their homes and on the pavements.

I asked the funeral director to do this because they had never asked him to do anything like it, but he didn't mind. I also asked him to place the photo on Lloyd's special bed at the service so everyone could see this brave little boy.

When we approached the church, there were hundreds of people. The inside of the church was to capacity with people, and some were even standing in the aisles.

As I stepped out of the family car, one of Lloyd's little friends came and gave me a teddy for Lloyd. And there was a ribbon on it that he had sewn "Lloyd Pike". I placed the teddy on top of Lloyd's special bed.

We held the handles of Lloyd's bed and lifted it onto a trolley, which we'd use to take Lloyd to the altar. I had Freesia flowers put all down the aisle so everybody could smell them when they entered the church.

They were also for family and friends to take with them after the service and place them on Lloyd's grave. We had Diana Ross singing "You Are Not Alone" as we entered the church, and when we left, the song playing was "I Hear Your Voice."

The service for Lloyd was beautiful; It couldn't have been any better. I wrote a letter for the curate to read about Lloyd's short but gorgeous life. It also thanked everyone for being a part of his life.

We had the songs "Morning Has Broken" and "All Creatures Great and Small." The curate spoke many beautiful words, accompanied by a message from Lloyd, which touched everyone.

Ty Hafan, Children's Hospice, kindly produced the order of service booklets, which had a gorgeous photograph of Lloyd on the front and a glitter teddy bear on the back. The service booklets were beautiful.

When Lloyd's special bed stood high on the altar, the bright sun shone through the stained window onto Lloyd's picture, and it amazed everyone in the church. I knew it was God because it had been raining all day, and suddenly the sun shone.

We then left for the cemetery, and as we drove through the cemetery gates, we turned right. We will bury Lloyd in a beautiful place, by the side of a wall and under a tree with a gorgeous blossom.

The bearers and I found it hard to lower Lloyd's special bed into the grave. It is the hardest thing we have ever had to do. The curate said some beautiful words, and everybody placed the Freesias from the church on Lloyd's special bed. I had a bouquet of Freesias made for me to carry and smell throughout the ceremony; I placed these on his unique bed.

The Ty Hafan nurses sprinkled glitter all over his unique bed, and I released ten helium balloons into the sky. We all watched them go higher and higher until they disappeared.

I said goodbye to Lloyd's friends, returned to his graveside and said, "I love you, and this is not goodbye. It is the start of a new life, and you will always be in my heart and thoughts every second of every day of my life, and we will love each other eternally."

Then, it was time for me to go.

We invited everyone back to The Star Inn for refreshments, and they served a buffet for family and friends.

Back at the pub, I had a cushion of flowers made, and we placed it in the seat where Lloyd always sat and put his photograph on the mantelpiece. It saddens me to be there without Lloyd in person, but I knew he was there in spirit.

The Ty Hafan nurses were at the Star Inn with my family and friends, and it saddened me that I had to go home without Lloyd. The thought of this was unbearable.

Before leaving The Star Inn for home, I needed to do something for Lloyd, something he loved doing. And that was to ring the bell for the last orders. So I took his photograph to the bar, and we rang the bell together.

The Star Inn has a photograph of Lloyd and me dressed up: me as a hippy and Lloyd as David Bowie at a fancy dress party. They have also hung a plaque under the photo, which says, "In Memory Of Lloyd." They have hung it just above his seat. When I got home, all I could do was cry. I didn't want to during the day because I always promised Lloyd I wouldn't in front of him.

On the day they diagnosed him, I cried, and Lloyd said, "I never want to see you cry again, Mum."

So, I needed to be brave at his funeral, but when I got home, it was time for me to break my heart, crying.

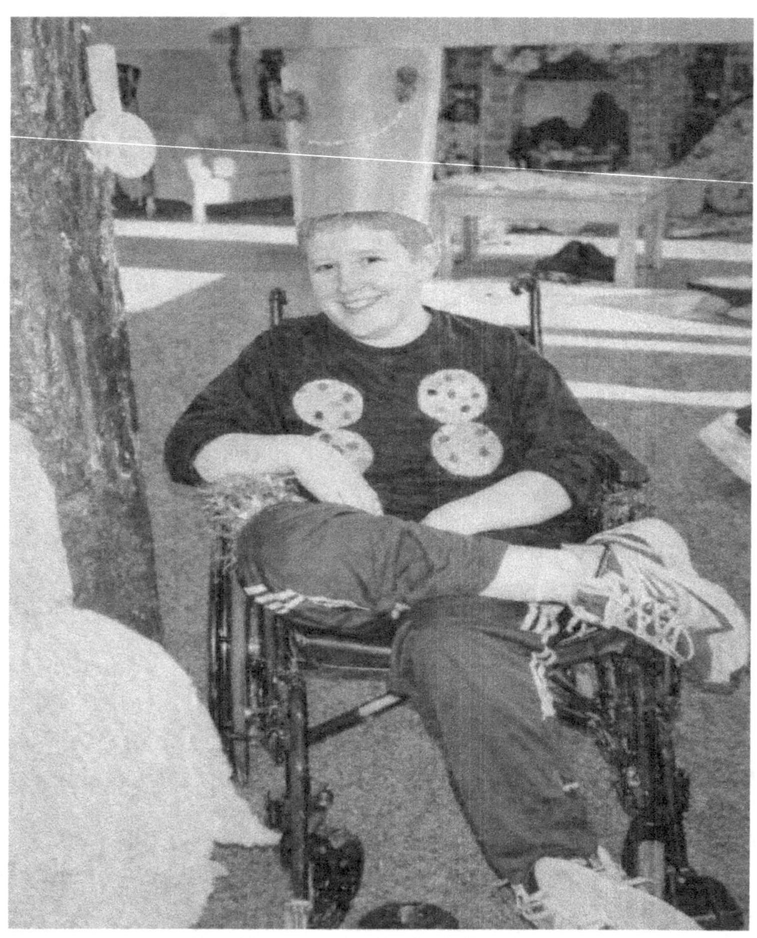

My Brave Little Soldier.

Chapter Twelve

Life After Life.

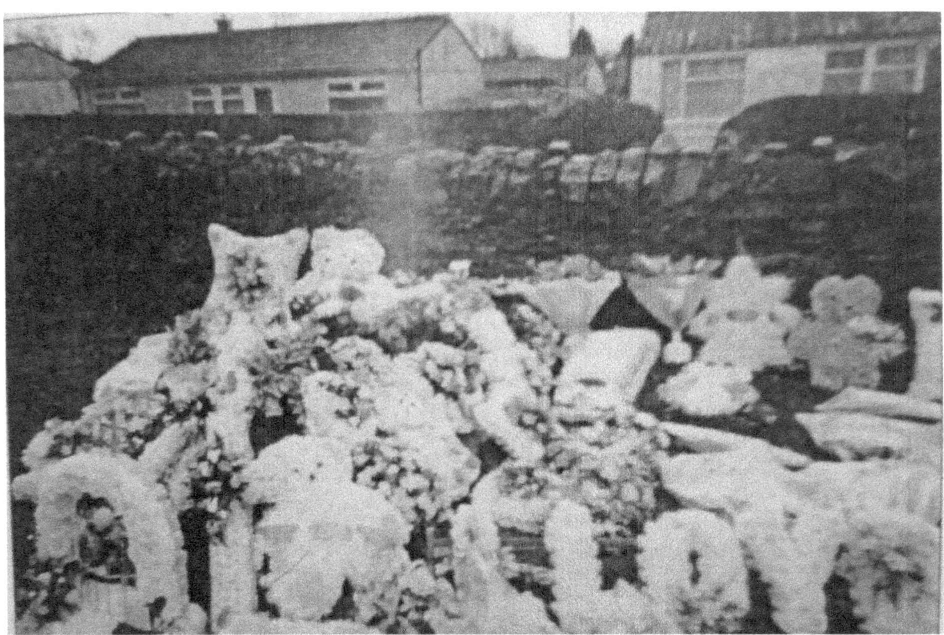

Friday, the 18 January 2002. Today, Lloyd's father and I visited the cemetery to look at all the floral tributes. There are hundreds. I wanted to use all the films in my camera to take photos of the flowers, to preserve them forever.

I will never use my camera or camcorder again because I only want to keep them as a memory of Lloyd. When I received the film back the next day from the developers, I noticed something on one photograph of Lloyd's flowers.

I believe it is Lloyd's spirit. I asked a photographer friend if there was an explanation for the light at the head of Lloyd's grave. He said he couldn't understand what it could be.

I go to the cemetery every day, and I always put flowers for my beautiful boy. Also, I will release balloons on special occasions.

I have chosen the perfect headstone for Lloyd's special place: it's a teddy bear, and I will have Lloyd's famous picture on the front put into an oval frame.

At this moment, I feel my life has ended, and I have nothing more to live for. I am alone, and although I have a wonderful family and friends, and my partner has always stood by me, my life has gone by.

All I have are my beautiful memories with hours of videos of Lloyd from his early life, which I watch because I need to see and hear him. I'm unable to watch TV, only Lloyd's videos.

I have 2,500 photographs of my Lloyd, mostly in albums and many more on the walls around our home. It's like Lloyd's gallery. The pictures are beautiful, and when you walk into our house, you can feel Lloyd's presence.

For those of you who have lost a loved one, you will know how I feel, especially when it concerns a child, but what keeps me going is that I believe there is a life afterlife.

I have proof of this, and I promise I won't lie. I have written this book to help others who may go through something similar. It has been hard writing it and living it all over again, but I hope, with all my heart, there is a message in here to help someone somewhere in the world.

Several days after Lloyd's funeral, I could smell Freesias, despite not having any in our home, and it was a strong smell. It has happened on three separate occasions.

I have had other proof. I always sleep in Lloyd's bedroom because I need to be close to him, and one evening, I had a nightmare. I have always had nightmares, and Lloyd would wake me, and while hugging me, he would say, "It's okay, mum. I'm here."

Tonight, I had a nightmare, and it frightened me. When I awoke, I realised I was alone and didn't have my Lloyd to hug and comfort me. Then suddenly, I could feel my back getting hugged and a hand on my hip. I knew it was Lloyd.

I never turned around because I knew I wouldn't see him, and I said, "Thank you, Lloyd. I love you," and then I went to sleep. It was unusual for me to go back to sleep after a nightmare, but I believed this had happened.

I have also heard Lloyd calling out to me, "MUM." So, if you believe and want it to happen, it will.

I have had many dreams about Lloyd, and they are beautiful. I feel him around me as if he is helping me, but I can't stop crying because he isn't with me. I miss caring for him, playing with him, and having our brilliant chats. He was my best friend and my loving son.

One morning, I had an unusual experience. I was lying on Lloyd's bed thinking of him when I could feel myself rising and looking down, and I could see my body on the bed. I thought I was dying, but I felt warm, relaxed and at peace. It overwhelmed me.

It was a beautiful feeling; I floated to a point and came back down. When this happened, I could feel my handheld and a kiss on my lips. Then, I settled back into my body. I am one hundred per cent sure it was my Lloyd.

Several days later, I went to see a medium, and the medium told me things only I knew, and no one could have known. I explained my encounter, and the medium said I had an out-of-body experience. They know this as Astral travel, and the medium told me I was privileged for it to have happened to me.

When I told her about my nightmare experience, she told me it was Lloyd and that if my spirit could leave my body to reach Lloyd, she was sure he would come to me when I needed him. But this is very rare.

I believe what I experienced was real, and I feel privileged that it happened. Our love for each other in this life will continue, even though we are apart. Which, I hope, will only be a short while.

I'm looking forward to the day we will be together again, but I need patience and to wait. I have a strong faith, and you require this. You also need to believe when you have experiences such as mine.

I have bought a book about Astral travel, and it explains my experience. The same thing has happened to thousands of other people.

It is difficult to carry on with your life when it has changed to such an enormous extent, but I need to carry on as best I can because my Lloyd fought as hard as he could for his life.

Lloyd had his pain, and now it's my turn.

But Lloyd had an unfamiliar physical pain, and one day, I will be able to control my pain, and that's the difference. I need to live on so Lloyd will live on in me.

To continue, you must set a target. Mine is raising money for Ty Hafan Children's Hospice. My brother-in-law, niece, and I are raising money through an activity they know as the Three-Peak Challenge.

They require us to climb three mountains in fifteen hours.

The mountains are Snowdon, Cader Idris, and Pen-Y-Fan in North Wales: 7,850 feet in fifteen hours, including travelling between them.

It's fabulous to have a target to meet, and practising in the Brecon Beacons gets me out of the house for several hours.

At present, after everything that has happened, I find it difficult to leave my home. I cannot get to terms with going out without Lloyd and pushing him around in his wheelchair.

But when I walk in the mountains, Lloyd and I are alone. And it's peaceful. I don't feel like being around crowds of people. I can't even go to my local shop.

I still have my front window blinds closed because it upsets me when I see children playing and coming home from school. Seeing other children still hurts, no matter their age. People tell me it will get better, but only time will tell.

Every night, when I go into Lloyd's bedroom, I look up to the sky and see the same star every time, and I know it is Lloyd's star. When I lie in bed, I talk to Lloyd, pray to God and thank him for all my wonderful family and friends.

And I also thank God for my special little boy, Lloyd, and ask him to send him to me in my dreams. I then say to my Lloyd, "Goodnight Lloyd, I love you, sweet dreams, God bless you," and then I sleep, hoping to dream about my Lloyd.

And the following day, I find it hard to rise from my bed and face another day without him. My family and friends can only imagine what it's like, but they will never know how I feel inside.

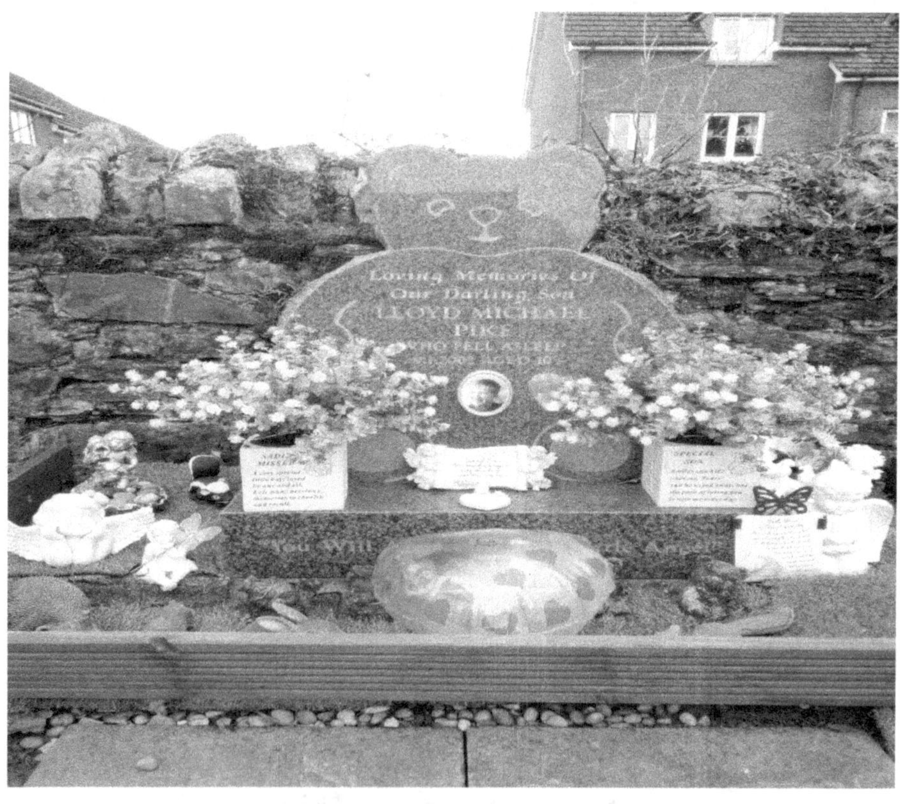

And this is the true story of Lloyd Michael Pike and those who share his beautiful memories with me. My long-term partner, Gareth, shared a massive part in our lives, and his son, Adam, was Lloyd's extra special friend. And Lloyd's dad, who loves him very much, and to our family and friends. We all love Lloyd and always will.

His memory will always be with us.

God bless Lloyd. You are all my dreams come true.

You gave so much to my heart and soul.

Thank you, Lloyd, from Mum.

The magic of your love has kept me going, and you have made ten years of my life so special. All I am, I owe to you, and I will love you forever.

XXXXXXXXXX

www.ingramcontent.com/pod-product-compliance
Lightning Source LLC
Chambersburg PA
CBHW081306250726
48662CB00008B/2420